© Copyright 2020 by Jo:

All rights reserve

The following book is created underneath to give information that is as accurate and reliable as conceivable. Regardless, purchasing this book can be viewed as agreeing to the fact that both the distributor and the author of this book are not the slightest bit specialists on the subjects examined inside and that any recommendations or proposals made thus are for entertainment purposes as it were. Professionals ought to be counseled as required before undertaking any of the actions embraced, therefore. This declaration is considered fair and valid by both the American Bar Association and the Committee of Publishers Association and is legally authoritative all through the United States.

Besides, the transmission, duplication, or proliferation of any of the following work, including specific information, will be viewed as an illegal act regardless if it is done electronically or in print. This stretches out to create a secondary or tertiary duplicate of the work or a recorded copy and is just allowed with a communicated composed permission from the distributor. All additional privileges held. The details in the following pages are broadly viewed as an honest and accurate account of facts. As such, any inattention, use, or abuse of the data being referred to by the reader will render any subsequent actions exclusively under their domain. There are no scenarios wherein the distributor or the original author of this work can be in any fashion considered liable for any hardship or damages that may happen after undertaking the information portrayed in this.

Additionally, the details in the following pages are planned uniquely for informational purposes and should along these lines be thought of as universal. As befitting its nature, it is introduced without assurance regarding its drawn-out validity or interval quality. Trademarks that are referenced are managed without composed permission and cannot be viewed as support from the trademark holder.

CARB CYCLING FOR BEGINNERS

100 Approved Recipes and Exercises to Lose Weight, Burn Fat and Get in Shape in 30 Days

BY

Joan DeCarli

TABLE OF CONTENTS

INTRODUCTION. 1

CHAPTER ONE; CARB CYCLING..3
- WHAT ARE MACRONUTRIENTS? 3
- WHERE DO CALORIES COME FROM?...4
- WHAT DO THE MACROS DO? 5
- WHERE DO MACROS COME FROM?..6
- BEST PROTEIN SOURCES 8
- BEST CARBOHYDRATE SOURCES..9
- BEST FAT SOURCES...9
- FIBER'S ROLE IN COUNTING CARBS..9
- WHAT CARB CYCLING IS NOT 11
- THE BASICS: HIGH-CARB DAYS AND LOW-CARB DAYS..........................11
- HIGH-CARB DAYS 11
- LOW-CARB DAYS 12
- HOW THE BODY LOSES FAT 12
- TOTAL FOOD INTAKE IS WHAT MATTERS...13
- COUNTING CALORIES WITH CARB CYCLING 14

CHAPTER TWO; THE BENEFITS OF CYCLING YOUR CARBOHYDRATE INTAKE 16
- HOW CARBOHYDRATES IMPACT YOUR BODY 16
- CONSTRUCT A DEFICIT WITH BOTH NUTRITION AND EXERCISE 24
- GETTING A CHARGE OUT OF THE FOODS YOU LIKE—IN MODERATION! 26

CHAPTER THREE; HOW TO GET STARTED 28
- TIPS AND TRICKS TO MAXIMIZE YOUR RESULTS....................................38

CHAPTER FOUR ADVANCED CARB CYCLING STRATEGIES 40
- ADDING EXERCISE 40
- ENDURANCE TRAINING VERSUS STRENGTH TRAINING 41
- STARTING AN ENDURANCE TRAINING PROGRAM 42
- CYCLING CARBS AROUND YOUR WORKOUTS 44
- BREAKING THROUGH FAT-LOSS PLATEAUS 45
- IS HIIT TRAINING, OR INTERVAL TRAINING, BENEFICIAL? 45
- STRENGTH TRAINING WORKOUTS 46
- SAMPLE HOME WORKOUTS 47
- FULL-BODY BEGINNER'S WORKOUT..48
- INTERMEDIATE WORKOUT 48
- CHEST AREA WORKOUT 49
- LOWER-BODY WORKOUT...49

  Cycling Carbs Around Your Workouts 50
  Staggered Carb Cycling 50
  The Weekly Depletion and Re-Feed 51
  Carb Back-Loading 53

CHAPTER FIVE; THE MAINTENANCE PHASE 54
  Do You Need to Carb Cycle Forever? 54
  Transitioning to a "Normal" Eating Style 56
  The Importance of Reverse Dieting 56
  Carb Cycling for Maintenance and forever 58
  Intuitive Eating versus Carb Cycling 60
  Working in High-Carb Days Without Gaining Fat 61

CHAPTER SIX; SAMPLE MEAL PLANS WITH RECIPES 63
  Sample Meal Plans 64
  Nutrient-Rich Vegetables 65
  Carbohydrates approved for Flexible Carb-Cycling Diet 67
  High-Carbohydrate Day 67
  High-fiber natural products approved for Flexible Carb-Cycling Diet 68
  Low-Carbohydrate Day 68
  Rules for No-Carb Days 69
  Days Leading up to Your Event 70

CHAPTER SEVEN; RECIPES, BREAKFAST 71
  1. Greek Egg Scramble 71
  2. Southwestern Omelet 72
  3. Chocolate Banana Protein Pancakes 74
  4. Apple Cinnamon Oatmeal 75
  5. High-Protein French Toast 76
  6. Egg White Protein Bites 78
  7. Power Wrap 79
  8. Two-Minute Chocolate Strawberry Protein Bowl 80
  9. Protein Scramble Bowl 82
  10. Low-Calorie Bacon, Egg, and Cheese 83
  11. Vanilla Raspberry Protein Fluff 84
  12. Berries and Cream Parfait 86
  12. Spinach, Red Onion, and Mushroom Frittata 87
  13. Huevos Rancheros 89
  14. Basic Sweet Potato Pancakes 91
  15. Clean Protein Power Bars 93
  16. Homemade Scallion Hash Brown Cakes 95

CHAPTER EIGHT; LUNCH 98
  17. Shrimp Stir-Fry 98

  18. Slow-Cooked Chicken 99

19. TURKEY BURGERS..101
20. SPAGHETTI SQUASH CRAB BLEND..103
21. SPINACH, FETA, AND PESTO CHICKEN QUESADILLAS...........................104
22. LOW-FAT CHICKEN BACON RANCH SANDWICH....................................106
23. SIRLOIN CHOPPED SALAD...107
24. SOUTHWESTERN FAJITAS..108
26. CHICKEN NACHOS..111
27. HEALTHY FRIED RICE..112
28. LEMON-HERB GRILLED CHICKEN SALAD..113
29. PULLED CHICKEN BBQ SANDWICH..114
30. SAUSAGE AND SPICY EGGS...115
31. LENTIL SALAD..117
32. PORTOBELLO MUSHROOM SALAD WITH GORGONZOLA, PEPPERS, AND BACON..118
33. ASPARAGUS SALAD WITH HARD-BOILED EGG....................................120

CHAPTER NINE; DINNER: BEEF, PORK, AND POULTRY 122

34. BAKED BUFFALO CHICKEN STRIPS..122
35. UN-DRIED TOMATO STUFFED CHICKEN...123
36. CHICKEN AND BEAN BURRITO...124
37. TAMARIND POT ROAST..125
38. TERRIFIC TAMARIND..126
39. MUSTARD PECAN CHICKEN..127
40. PAPAYA PULLED PORK..128
41. PESTO PORK CHOPS...129
42. ARGENTINIAN STEAK...131
43. LEAN MEAT BALLS...132
44. TUSCAN CHICKEN..134
45. LAGER CAN CHICKEN..135
46. STEAKHOUSE BLUE CHEESE BURGER..137
47. SPAGHETTI MARINARA WITH CHICKEN AND BASIL............................138
48. LEAN TURKEY MEATLOAF..140
49. MARINATED GRILLED TURKEY CUTLETS..142
50. GARLIC-STUDDED PORK ROAST...144

CHAPER TEN; DINNER: FISH AND SHELLFISH 146

51. DIJON TUNA...146
52. COCONUT GARLIC SHRIMP...147
53. SHRIMP-ORANGE KEBABS..148
54. SPINACH AND FETA SALMON...149
55. STUFFED SALMON FILETS..150
56. SALMON BURGERS...152
57. SUN-DRIED TOMATO TUNA...153
58. LEMON AND GARLIC COD FILETS..154
59. SHRIMP SCAMPI...155

60. FIRM PARMESAN FISH STICKS..156
61. FETA AND TUNA PASTA SALAD..157

62. FETA AND TUNA PASTA SALAD 158
63. HIGH-PROTEIN TUNA MELT 159
64. LEMON PEPPER TILAPIA 160
65. SHRIMP CEVICHE 161

CHAPTER ELEVEN; VEGETARIAN MAINS, SIDES, AND SALADS .163

66. VEGETARIAN CAKES 163
67. HIGH-PROTEIN SPREAD 164
68. BANANA OATMEAL 165
69. QUINOA BURRITOS 166
70. ZESTY PEANUT TEMPEH SALAD 167
71. BAKED EGGPLANT AND BELL PEPPER 168
72. ZUCCHINI OVEN FRIES 169
73. LEMON QUINOA 170
74. FRESH CORN, PEPPER, AND AVOCADO SALAD 171
75. SOUTHWESTERN BEET SLAW 173
76. BEAN SALAD WITH ORANGE VINAIGRETTE 174
77. BASIC AUTUMN SALAD 176
78. VEGETABLE-STUFFED POBLANO PEPPERS 177
79. PORTOBELLO TACOS 178

CHAPTER TWELVE; VEGAN MAINS, SIDES, AND SALADS 181

80. VEGETABLE STEW WITH CORNMEAL DUMPLINGS 181
81. RED BEANS AND RICE 183
82. MEDITERRANEAN CHICKPEA BAKE 184
83. SMALLER THAN EXPECTED VEGETABLE BURGERS 185
84. ARUGULA AND FENNEL SALAD WITH POMEGRANATE 187
84. APPLE COLESLAW 188
85. ROOT VEGETABLE SALAD 189
86. KALE AND SEA VEGETABLES WITH ORANGE-SESAME DRESSING 191
87. RED PEPPER AND FENNEL SALAD 192
88. CASHEW-ZUCCHINI SOUP 194
89. SAAG TOFU 196
90. RED ONION AND OLIVE FOCACCIA 197
91. SUMMER VEGETABLE TIAN 199
92. SWEET AND SPICY BRUSSELS SPROUTS 200
93. GARLICKY CHICKPEAS AND SPINACH 201

CHAPTER THIRTEEN PASTA 204

94. FARFALLE WITH CHICKEN AND PESTO 204
95. WHOLE-WHEAT PENNE WITH KALE AND CANNELLINI BEANS 205
96. BAKED RAVIOLI 206
97. BROCCOLI-BASIL PESTO AND PASTA 207

98. CHICKEN AND BROCCOLI FETTUCCINE 208
99. PEPPER, ONION, AND SHRIMP KEBABS 210

CHAPTER FOURTEEN; SOUPS 212
- 100. CORN AND BLACK BEAN CHILI 212
- 101. CREAMY CORN CHOWDER 213
- 102. PUMPKIN SOUP BASE 214
- 103. SWEET AND SPICY CARROT SOUP 215
- DESSERTS 217
- 104. PEANUT BUTTER PROTEIN COOKIES 217
- 105. OATMEAL PROTEIN COOKIES 218
- 106. PROTEIN CHEESECAKE 219
- 107. PEANUT BUTTER BANANA FROZEN GREEK YOGURT 220
- 108. CINNAMON-PEAR FROZEN YOGURT 220

CONCLUSION 222

INTRODUCTION.

In the world of dieting, there are innumerable choices and plans for you to follow. Many are based on extraordinary limitations, eliminating one food group or another. Some are based around the timing of meals, tallying calories or focuses, or simply eating "clean" foods. It is often overwhelming, and with so many alternatives, it's hard to know which is the best.

When you consider the number of other options and the fact that a large portion of them use overhyped stories and pictures in their marketing, you may be enticed to surrender all together simply, the best diet is the one you can adhere to. Any plan that has you eating less food than you need will assist you with losing fat. The difference is that some plans make this easy and fun, and some make it miserable.

One thing you want to understand is that you can't eat certain food because as soon as something is prohibited, chances are you'll crave it significantly more. Carbohydrate cycling is probably the easiest technique you can use to evacuate unwanted body fat. It takes a touch of planning, but the execution is extremely easy and painless. There are no limitations, as any food you appreciate can be made to fit in the plan. It's instinctive and makes sense once you learn a tad about how your body procedures and utilizations food. In addition to helping you lose fat, carbohydrate cycling can have an entire host of other benefits as well, something that not all diet plans can say.

This e-book will take you through the whole procedure, giving all of you the tools, you'll have to start your excursion and observe sustainable outcomes. You'll learn what carb cycling is and what it isn't. You'll learn about macronutrients, how your body utilizes the food you eat, and the impact practice has on your body. After reading, you'll realize how to plan for social occasions, vacations, or any other time you want to eat a lot of your favorite foods, without fixing all of your advancement. Finally, this book will show you how to make sense of how much food you ought to eat and how to set up a carb cycling plan that suits your life. Before the finish of the book, you will realize how to start your program and manipulate it as you go, and you'll have an entire pack of recipes to kick you off. It takes time, and results won't happen for the time being, but with a little patience and some hard work, you'll have the option to decrease your body fat levels and finally earn your dream body. Perhaps most importantly, this book will teach you what to do after reaching your initial goals on a diet. Most books teach you how to eat and work out to reach your goal, and end with the assumption that you'll get your dream body. Regardless of whether you do reach your goals, what comes after is simply as important, as returning immediately to your old habits is a surefire way to gain all the weight back. This plan will show how to transition from dieting to a maintenance mode that you can easily maintain forever.

CHAPTER ONE: CARB CYCLING

Carb cycling is a dietary method that allows you to advance your body arrangement by losing fat and building lean muscle, without the pressure of extraordinary food limitations or calorie checking. By strategically manipulating the number of carbohydrates you expend daily, it is easy to set up a fat-consuming environment in your body, which can be maintained easily and for significant periods.

What Are Macronutrients?

Before anything can be examined about carb cycling, it's important to characterize what exactly a carbohydrate is. Your body depends on food to live and utilizes the calories devoured through food to play out all the elements of daily living. All calories originate from macronutrients, which are carbohydrates, proteins, and fats. A calorie is a system of measurement used to portray the amount of energy gained from expending a certain food. Set up a fat-consuming environment in your body that can be maintained easily and for significant periods. **Macronutrients** are proteins, carbs, and fat. You can recall this because macro means large. Micronutrients, then again, while essential, don't have any calories. Micronutrients would incorporate vitamins, minerals, antioxidants, and different things found in food that don't have any calories.

Where Do Calories Come From?

When caloric values from food are calculated for labeling purposes, it is the macronutrients that are being measured. A gram of carbohydrate has 4 calories, a gram of protein has 4 calories, and a gram of fat has 9 calories. Vitamins and minerals, also called micronutrients, are essential to the ideal working of the human body but don't give any caloric value. So when you take a gander at a label, all that gets factored into the total calories are the protein, carb, and fat totals. These are recorded in grams, while different nutrients may be recorded in different measurements, or even percentages of your daily suggested intake.

You may be interested in how alcohol fits in. While it has both advantages and drawbacks, speaking carefully as far as calories, alcohol is a peculiarity. It has 7 calories for each gram, more than protein and carbs, but not exactly fat. However, it doesn't give any nutrients, so it is simply empty calories. Wine, brew, and sugary blended beverages will usually have carbohydrates as well, but pure alcohol just has alcohol calories.

A healthy diet will comprise of an appropriate balance of all three macronutrients, as all are essential for optimal living. You may have the option to get by with a low intake of one, but it's generally not going to have you feeling your best. For example, you can go significant periods with no carbohydrate intake, as long as protein and fat intake are adequate. Still, your energy levels and recuperation from physical activity will endure. If you go low-fat for extensive periods, you can experience the ill effects of all sorts of negative hormonal impacts, for example, decreased testosterone in the two people, and brought down estrogen in ladies. Low testosterone and estrogen can lead to a decrease in sex drive, lower energy, and higher body fat to lean mass ratio.

What Do the Macros Do?

Proteins are utilized to revamp many different cells in the body, and advantage skin, hair, fingernails, muscle development, and many different capacities. You may have heard that you need protein to assemble muscle, and this is valid, which makes it easy to recollect that you need protein to repair and fabricate pretty much anything in your body. Proteins are the structure squares of the body. Fats are generally slower to process, give a satiating, or craving blunting, impact, and are necessary for optimal hormonal profiles. There are many misinterpretations about fat, and many diets recommend eating as minimal fat as conceivable, but this isn't smart or healthy. Of course, some sorts of fats are superior to other people, but you need fat to live, and the correct fats are extremely beneficial to your body. During times of limited carbohydrate intake, the fat turns out to be considered increasingly important to flexibly energy.

Carbohydrates are a fascinating macronutrient. While not technically necessary to get by—as your body can break down protein and convert it into a type of glucose, which is what carbohydrates are made of—they give a fast-processing, readily available energy source. When separated into glucose, they elevate glucose levels and give energy to the body, and are utilized during higher-force activities, for example, exercise, sports, or physical occupations. Some individuals will reveal to you that carbohydrates are essential to staying alive since your brain needs glucose to work. However, through a cool little procedure called gluconeogenesis, or the transformation of protein to carbs, your body can make glucose without carbs. It takes some time, and it's not ideal, but it tends to be finished.

As far as body organization, no single macronutrient is the way to reaching your goal, and no macronutrient alone is a replacement for fat. You can devour any food in abundance and gain fat. To work at optimal levels, you ought to eat protein, carbs, and fat in the best possible amounts, and avoid eliminating any one of those nutrients.

Identifying Carbohydrates, Proteins, and Fats Now that the macronutrients have been characterized, it's important to have the option to identify what sorts of foods each originates from. You may realize that you have to eat high-protein foods, but you also need to comprehend what those foods are. Many entire food sources will predominantly be one macronutrient or the other, with some protein sources containing fat as well. With profoundly handled foods, it isn't easy to recognize what will be what, so it's important to check the nourishment label as you shop and plan for your meals.

Where Do Macros Come From?

Carbohydrates are found in starchy food sources, natural products, and vegetables. Normal sources incorporate potatoes, rice, and high-sugar natural products, for example, bananas, grapes, and mangos. To a lesser degree, carbohydrates are also found in vegetables, although frequently in much lower quantities. The most noteworthy carbohydrate levels are found in handled sugary food, for example, cereal, bread, rice, pasta, crackers, dried organic product, and soda pops. Protein is something to pay special attention to. A total protein consists of twenty different amino acids, all of which have varying jobs in the body. The more kinds of amino acids a protein contains, the more complete it is thought of. The greater part of the tissue in your body is made out of amino acids, which are the structure squares of protein and your body, so it's important to get adequate amounts of all twenty amino acids. Not all food sources contain all twenty of these amino acids, so the more amino a protein has, the more "complete" it is thought of. Among those amino acids are essential amino acids, which are the amino acids your body needs, but cannot deliver itself. You should get these essential amino acids by consuming protein sources. The best wellsprings of complete protein are eggs, chicken, fish, hamburger, pork, and dairy items. While a couple of plant sources, like beans and nuts, may contain trace amounts of protein, they frequently don't have all twenty amino acids. If you are following a vegetarian diet, you may have to join several plant sources to obtain all twenty amino acids, since you won't get them from meat sources.

Fats are most generally found in nuts, avocados, oils, and high-fat protein sources, for example, salmon, egg yolks, certain cuts of red meat, fattier cuts of pork, and dairy items, for example, butter and cheddar. Many prepared foods you see at the store will also be high in fat. As recently mentioned, fat is high in calories, therefore high-fat foods will have significantly more significant calorie checks. Never forget that while fat is essential for living, a gram of fat will have over more than the calories of a gram of protein or carbohydrate, so you would prefer not to consume boundless amounts of fat. As you start thinking about what sorts of foods you want to keep in the house, here is a rundown of the best food hotspots for each macronutrient. When consumed regularly, these foods flexibly a lot of good micronutrients and antioxidants and give a variety of nutrients to your body. While different foods are acceptable, obviously, but the ones recorded here will give healthy, nutritious hotspots for your macronutrients, and ought to be the foundation of the greater part of your meals.

Antioxidants help shield the body from free radicals, which can damage the healthy cells in your body. Free radicals can be created by your body's regular capacity, upsetting situations, or by an introduction to environmental toxins, for example, contamination, smoke, and herbicides. Antioxidants neutralize the threat of the free radicals by affecting their electrical charge, keeping them from damaging different cells.

Best Protein Sources:
- Boneless, skinless chicken breast
- Whole eggs/egg whites
- Lean turkey breast or ground turkey

- Low-fat fish
- Low-fat red meat
- Low-fat cottage cheddar

Best Carbohydrate Sources:

- Potatoes (any shading)
- Rice
- Fruits and vegetables, in a variety of hues
- Oats

Best Fat Sources:

- Nuts
- Avocados
- Coconut oil
- High-fat cuts of red meat
- High-fat fish
- Whole eggs

Fiber's Role in Counting Carbs

It is also necessary to characterize fiber, as many different brands and companies remember it in different ways. Fiber is a part of certain carbohydrates that generally comprises a lot of denser material. Your body has a harder time processing fiber, so if you consume higher amounts of fiber, you will likely notice that you stay full more. As far as health benefits, fiber can improve digestion, glucose levels, recurrence of solid discharges, and is generally useful to remember for your diet. Because fiber is so thick and hard to process, many labeling or diet systems expel fiber from the total carbohydrate check. Thus, a food with 20 grams of carbohydrate and 5 grams of fiber may list "15 net carbs" on the label because the 5 grams of fiber isn't processed as fast as starchy carbs. However, it is as still important to take a look at total carbs, as fiber doesn't cancel them out, contrary to what some labels would have you accept. Adding fiber powder to frozen yogurt, for example, would not nullify the impacts of the high sugar levels found in the desert. If this worked, you could basically carry around a fiber supplement and consume it with all your carbs to cancel them out, which unfortunately would not work well. You always have to take a gander at the total carbohydrates.

If you've read about carbohydrates at any point, you may be familiar with the glycemic list. The glycemic file is a measure of how fast carbohydrates raise glucose levels. Exceptionally prepared carbs have a high glycemic record, as they spike your glucose rapidly. Carbs high in fiber have a much lower number on the glycemic record, which is why they are regularly suggested—you want stable glucose levels, not shoots all over all day. Stringy food sources incorporate green leafy vegetables, some organic products, and entire grain carbohydrate sources, for example, oatmeal. It is also conceivable to add fiber supplements to a diet if the diet doesn't give adequate fiber; however, you should always consult a healthcare professional before taking any dietary supplements. When following the plans in this book, always count up total carbohydrates; don't subtract fiber from the total.

What Carb Cycling Is Not

There are many popular diets out there, and many are based around the idea that carbs make you fat, this belief has to be eliminated. It doesn't make a difference if you eat boundless amounts of fat and protein, according to these diets, because carbs are the genuine enemy. This isn't accurate. Carbohydrate cycling is a way of eating that allows you to have varying carb intakes on different days of the week. It's anything but an elimination diet, where carbs are banned in all structures inconclusively. It is also not a low-fat diet—on low-carb days, fat may be very high to reach the necessary caloric intake level. Carb levels fluctuate when utilizing cycling, versus an all-or-nothing approach that has been made popular by so many different diets.

The Basics: High-Carb Days and Low-Carb Days

The most basic type of carb cycling is to have two degrees of carbohydrate intake: high and low. Different strategies will be detailed later on, with varying daily degrees of carbohydrate intake, but for now, just high and low days will be discussed.

High-Carb Days

On higher-carb days, carb sources will incorporate rice, pasta, organic product, and potatoes—tradition-starchy carbohydrate sources. High-carb days should fall on days with high physical activity. If physical activity is not a normal daily schedule, at that point, high-carb days should be set around personal inclination, for example, on the week-finishes to allow for socially guilty pleasures. On higher-carb days, protein intake should generally stay the same, with an emphasis on lower-fat sources. Since carb intake is higher, total calories will also increase, so to counterbalance this; total fat should be brought down. Calories must be controlled for weight misfortune to happen, so individuals who use carb cycling to lose fat ought to make sure always to keep total calories generally the same each day.

Low-Carb Days

On low-carb days, carb intake ought to be set low. Most meals should be made up of proteins and vegetables, with the daily carb intake being constrained to the trace carbs in vegetables and maybe one serving of a natural product. It's important to avoid drinking anything with unreasonable amounts of carbs, as this can defeat the purpose of a low-carb day. Similarly, as with the high-carb day, fat will be adjusted. On this kind of day, however, fat intake should increase, since carbs are decreased.

How the Body Loses Fat

To understand why this works, and why some of the guidelines that will be laid out are necessary, it's important to initially have a general understanding of how fat misfortune and gain happen in the body. There are so many gossipy tidbits about the fat misfortune that simply aren't accurate. Fat doesn't simply dissolve away or transform into muscle, and your body probably won't store pounds of fat off of one major meal. Body fat is essentially energy that has been stored away. As referenced earlier, food is measured in calories, a unit of measurement to depict the amount of energy gained from that food. All daily activities of living, in addition to any physical activity, utilize these calories. If you are moving around all day, you'll consume more calories than if you sat as the day progressed. Similarly, if a diet gives a larger number of calories than required, your body will hope to store the abundance as energy in muscle, or as adipose tissue, the actual fat on the body.

Total Food Intake Is What Matters

When you are in a caloric surplus, the weight will be gained, as you are eating more calories than your body can utilize. If someone is hoping to add muscle and is following a legitimate workout program, this may be wanted. However, for fat loss, there must be a caloric deficit—that is, eating fewer calories than you consume. The primary law of thermodynamics applies here: energy cannot be created or destroyed, just transformed. If your body uses a greater number of calories than it takes in, it has to get the energy from somewhere, and put away fat is an ideal place. If you eat such a large number of calories, you'll gain body fat. This is why a caloric shortfall causes fat misfortune and absolutely should be in place for fat misfortune to happen. Without this caloric deficiency, you cannot diminish body fat. There are no mystery workouts, pills, magic foods, or anything else that can get around this standard. Some diets will attempt as far as possible fat or carbohydrate intake. The reason this is successful is that by evacuating those food groups, a caloric deficit is created. However, there is nothing naturally malicious about any food group; all that matters at long last is maintaining a caloric shortage.

Many individuals accept that sweating abundantly during a workout means you are losing fat. If you notice that you are several pounds lighter after a workout, it's conceivable some of that was fat, but the chances are that the majority of that weight was water lost through sweating, not actual fat loss. Never forget to rehydrate yourself and drink a lot of liquids after any activity where you are heavily sweating. When your body reaches where energy output is greater than in-take, it will start to metabolize, or break down and use body fat. The fat cells are transported to the cells of our bodies that will break them down for energy, or "consume" them. In this way, the body breaks down fat and transports it to be utilized for energy. This energy is then utilized for calorie-consuming activities, with the waste being evacuated through sweat, pee, and exhaling of breath.

Counting Calories with Carb Cycling

You realize that you should control total calories to lose body fat. However, this doesn't really mean you have to tally them each day. While this may be a smart move most of the time, contingent upon your degree of order, you may have the option to see great outcomes without tallying calories **regularly**. Just by the nature of limiting carbs on certain days, chances are you are creating an adequate caloric shortage, at least if you have a better than average amount of fat to lose. If your food decisions generally stay the same, with brought down carbs on certain days, you shouldn't have an excess of difficulty losing fat, at least initially. However, if you wind up eating foods, you wouldn't normally eat, especially high-fat foods, you may end up in a tough situation.

There is nothing wrong with eating high-fat foods in moderation, since you despite everything, make sure you aren't overshooting your total daily calorie goal. For example, if your protein sources stay the same and add a couple of extra eggs, or an avocado, on your low-carb day, you'll probably be okay. However, if you start eating eggs, bacon, steak, handfuls of nuts all day—you may be eating a lot of fat.

Later on in this book, you'll learn how to make sense of how many calories you ought to eat to maintain or get thinner, but for the time being, simply realize that it isn't necessary to count calories if you have the self-control to avoid high-fat foods on your low-carb days. Start without tallying. Mindfully follow the plans that will come later in the book, and see what happens. If you discover you don't see the outcomes you want, you may have to start checking calories for some time.

Chapter Two; The Benefits Of Cycling Your Carbohydrate Intake

There are many advantages of cycling your carbohydrate intake past just improving your rate of fat loss. From helping control your appetite and energy levels to improving mental concentration and in any event, improving your hormonal balance, carbohydrate cycling can do a lot of great things for your body. It's important to first understand what happens when you eat carbohydrates, as far as digestion and the resulting impacts. Then you can completely understand and actualize the advantages of cycling.

How Carbohydrates Impact Your Body

You already realize what carbohydrates are and where they come from. Now it's an ideal opportunity to understand what happens to them once they are consumed. The procedure starts with digestion. During the digestion phase, your body works to break down the carbohydrates into single particles of glucose. Contingent upon the kind of carbohydrate, this breakdown may be fast or moderate. Straightforward carbohydrates will be processed more rapidly than complex carbohydrates, as they can be separated faster, which is an important point to recall moving for-ward.

Glucose is the substance that will be referenced frequently here, as it is the body's favored source of energy. It is most normally found in grains, potatoes, rice, and other starchy foods. However, fundamentally the same as a particle called fructose, discovered mainly in organic products, has a similar impact on glucose and is also immediately processed. So while the natural product doesn't have glucose, it breaks down into fructose, nearly the same thing. As part of the digestion procedure, the glucose is next absorbed into the bloodstream, where it very well may be carried around to places that need it, or it could be put away in adipose tissue (body fat cells) for later use. Eating a large portion of carbohydrates will elevate your glucose levels, with straightforward carbohydrates bringing about a fast increase and complex carbohydrates, bringing about a slower, progressively stable increase. While it's not necessarily bad to have high glucose currently, chronically high glucose can increase one's risk of turning out to be pre-diabetic or creating diabetes later in life.

Ideally, glucose ought to be kept as stable as possible. If it's excessively low, you'll feel tired and can get unsteady or lightheaded, and if it gets too high too rapidly, you'll experience an energy surge followed by a sharp crash, which can make you feel worn out and moody.

Issues with High Carbohydrate Intake

In light of glucose is elevated, your body will look to process the glucose as quickly as possible. When your body senses an elevation in glucose, it signals the pancreas release insulin, which will help clear the blood of glucose and get it put away appropriately. Insulin encourages your body to store nutrients that are in the bloodstream. Whether it's glucose from carbohydrates, amino acids from proteins, or fatty acids, your body will hope to move these to storage when insulin is released. Nutrients can be put away in muscles or various organs to recharge their stores, but if those stores are full, and the nutrients won't be stored for energy, they will be put away as fat tissue. If you are eating high-sugar foods regularly, your body should utilize more insulin.

The more you have to utilize insulin to bring down glucose levels, the less compelling it turns out to be, almost like building up a tolerance for caffeine, which becomes less successful with constant use, requiring increasingly more to get the ideal impact. At the point when you have chronically elevated glucose, your body requires greater amounts of insulin to handle the sugar load, which after some time, can increase your risk of creating type 2 diabetes. In this condition, your body can't deliver enough insulin to control glucose, causing your blood sugar levels to ascend excessively high. With type 2 diabetes, you lose your insulin sensitivity, meaning you need more insulin increasingly to do the same amount of work. Eventually, your pancreas just can't deliver enough insulin to keep up. In type 1 diabetes, a condition you are brought into the world with, your body just doesn't create insulin, so you'll have to infuse it regularly or have an insulin siphon that automatically keeps insulin in your system at all occasions.

Carbohydrate cycling can help improve your insulin sensitivity; By using significant stretches of lower carbohydrate intake, you can allow your body to reset itself and learn to use insulin appropriately again. Improved insulin sensitivity is only one of the many health advantages of cycling your carbohydrate intake, in addition to helping your body use carbohydrates more effectively rather than putting them away as fat. Note that a lot of this negative glucose spiking can be negated by picking intricate, high-fiber carbs and spreading them over some time. It's as yet a great idea to cycle your carbohydrate intake on a day-to-day basis, as the glucose will eventually make it to your bloodstream regardless of the source. Still, high-fiber, complex carbs can diminish the number of fast glucose spikes. The fast spikes and resulting drops in glucose that originate from eating straightforward carbs can cause fatigue, hunger, mood swings, headaches, and other negative impacts, so it's ideal to avoid this as much as conceivable.

Stabilizing Blood Sugar and Losing Fat; Stabilizing your glucose will greatly aid you in your endeavors to lose fat. The greater part of the accompanying information will apply to your higher-carbohydrate days, where you will be sure to be taking in carbs for the day, but it's valuable information to know. If your carbs are profoundly handled, basic sources, you may endure glucose crashes that originate from a high amounts of prepared carbs. These crashes leave you feeling exceptionally cranky and hungry. If you've eaten a bag of candy or a donut or two, you'll realize that it doesn't keep you anywhere near as full as a bowl of oatmeal, even though the total carbohydrate check may be the same. When attempting to diet and exercise self-control, the last thing you need is to feel cranky and hungry from a glucose crash. Ultimately, total calories are all that matter when losing fat, but if you can keep your energy levels, mood, and yearning leveled out, you'll have a lot easier time sticking to a plan.

Fruits and vegetables have carbohydrates, but aren't they expected to be healthy? Leafy foods are a phenomenal source of a variety of vitamins and minerals that you require for optimal health, so indeed, they are healthy for you. With vegetables, you'll usually be getting a lot of fiber as well, especially with many kinds of greens, so you shouldn't stress over those. While healthy, organic products are also brimming with sugar, so be careful with them if you're stressed over glucose. It's natural sugar, but sugar in any case, and it can cause glucose spikes if consumed in large quantities. As a symptom of attempting to control your glucose levels, you'll probably be decreasing your calories, and wind up accelerating your fat loss endeavors. By stabilizing your glucose, you'll improve your mood and diminish your cravings. This is generally achieved by decreasing your basic carbohydrate intake—the two have a synergistic relationship that works to assist you with staying on your plan. You'll eat less prepared carbs, have better energy and mood for the day, and experience fewer appetite cravings caused by glucose drops.

Boosting Mental Clarity; Focus, and Energy Stabilizing glucose and lessening the good and bad times associated with carbohydrate intake generally bring about better mental work. This may not appear as though a major factor when you are thinking about starting a diet, but once the negative manifestations start to come out, you'll know exactly why they can make dieting miserable.

Steady glucose levels will allow you to feel happier and less cranky when dieting, give you sustained energy all day and help you avoid the brain haze you can regularly feel from limited carbs and/or fatigue. Carbohydrates do give energy to the body, and you will utilize glucose for many daily living elements, so it's important to have some in your body. The goal is to have sustained energy all day; however, not large surges of energy followed by crashes, which can make you want to look for that surge again. If you eat a major, sugary breakfast, for example, a bagel and natural product, you'll probably see a crash later in your workday, when you feel drained, unable to center, hungry, and moody. You don't want that. If you pick high-fiber, entire food carb sources, and spread them out for the day, you'll no doubt feel full more, feel stimulated for the day, and feel alert and centered.

Note that it may take a brief period to adapt to fewer carbohydrates or a decrease in the sugary ones. If you are used to eating a lot of carbs each day, the first occasion when you attempt to diminish or eliminate them, you may feel cranky, and feel that your brain is foggy—meaning that it appears to be harder to center and procedure things—and you may feel distracted and agitated. This timeframe may be unpleasant, but eventually, your body will make sense that it's not getting high portions of sugar spikes for the day, and it will stabilize and adjust to your new eating habits. Have some patience and trust the procedure. You'll be in an ideal situation over the long haul.

Outsmarting Hunger and Staying on Track; Appetite is a dubious thing. In general, there are two main sorts of appetite: emotional craving and physical yearning. Emotional craving is normal and hard to perceive. You may wind up feeling hungry if you are exhausted, vexed, pushed, happy, craving something there are many triggers for emotional appetite. Physical yearning is your body revealing to you; it needs nutrients, not a straightforward craving. Physical yearning can't be controlled; after all, if you go an extended period without eating, your body will rush to tell you. While progressively normal for many, emotional craving is also the most exceedingly awful kind, as you will be enticed to eat all sorts of food you needn't bother with. It's important to learn how to perceive emotional appetite, and learn what you can never really control. There are a couple of basic deceives you can use to assist you with learning to feel the difference between emotional yearning and physical appetite. The first is to just go quite a while without eating one day—attempt to hold off until mid-afternoon, supper, or as long as you can. Those afternoon hours will be extreme, and you'll see physical indications of yearning that won't leave. It's ideal to do this when you can stay occupied, so you aren't considering food—and don't stress, it's safe to do as long as you drink a lot of water. In addition to the fact that this is a great exercise in self-control, but you'll learn what genuine physical yearning feels like.

Improving Your Hormonal Profile; Managing your carbohydrate intake can have positive impacts on your hormonal profile as well, especially if it leads to a decrease in body fat. As discussed earlier, insulin management is important for an entire host of things. Controlling carbohydrate intake can also be beneficial to sex hormone creation, mainly testosterone and estrogen. If you are an after a diet plan that suggests a diminished carbohydrate intake, you will probably be eating increasingly healthy fats as part of the plan, to make up for the caloric deficiency created from expelling the carbs. Hormonal working is unpredictable, but increasing your healthy dietary fat intake and stabilizing glucose can help bolster healthy hormone levels in the two people.

Building a Caloric Deficit for Fat Loss; To lower body fat levels, you should be in a caloric deficiency. It is impossible to avoid this. Everybody's metabolism is different, so everybody has different caloric needs, but if you are not consuming a higher number of calories than you are eating, you won't have the option to lose fat. Several strategies can be utilized to get yourself into the required caloric deficit for weight misfortune.

Create a Caloric Deficit with Food; The least difficult way to create a caloric deficiency is to eat less food. If you are taking in 2,500 calories per day, diminishing your intake to 2,000 is a great place to start and should be truly manageable. It's not all that much, and by replacing some high-calorie foods with some lower-calorie, all the more filling foods, such as sinewy vegetables and lean proteins, you ought to have the option to control your craving as well.

If you don't have time to work out, don't have the foggiest idea how, or simply want a basic way to start your fat-misfortune venture, the initial step should always be just to eat less food.

Manufacture a Caloric Deficit with Exercise; The subsequent way to create a caloric shortfall is by increasing your physical activity. All life elements use calories for energy, from getting up and making breakfast to going for a run, and everything in the middle. By increasing your energy yield each day, you can help create a shortage and consume more calories. The one issue with utilizing activity to create a deficiency is attempting to make sense of how many calories you are consuming. Everyone is different, so using calories-consumed calculators and various tools may not be the most accurate strategy. It's a start, but it won't be great. It's also important to take note of that as you show signs of improvement at things, or increasingly proficient, it takes less energy to play out the action. You may take a long walk around the area and feel exhausted, but if you do this same walk each day, after half a month, you'll be consuming many fewer calories than when you started. Rather than attempt to calculate how many calories you consumed when you accomplish something, simply attempt to move all the more consistently and appreciate the procedure, realizing you are taking care of your body and making it work better.

Construct a Deficit with Both Nutrition and Exercise

The most productive way to create the caloric shortage expected to lose fat is to utilize both diet and exercise to reach your goals. You could get by with only either, but since a healthy diet and regular exercise have so many health benefits, there is no reason to leave one on the table. The two will work together to make you stronger and healthier and assist you with reaching your weight-misfortune goals. By having a regular, challenging activity plan in place, making a push to move more at whatever point you can. Following a healthy meal plan that gives you the appropriate amount of calories for your goals, be sure you are doing your absolute best to set yourself up for success. If you are regularly practicing, be careful not to eat extra food to make available, thinking you earned it. A lively 30-minute workout may consume 250–300 calories, which is a great accomplishment. Still, it's all too easy to think about eating those calories directly back up, even with something that may appear healthy. If you are regularly practicing, you will have the option to eat more overall than if you were sedentary, but be smart about it. On the other side, if you overeat, don't attempt to consume practice and rebuff yourself; you'll be miserable. Simply lower your calories for the following, not many days, and get directly back on track. At long last, all that matters is creating a steady caloric shortage. Some weeks you'll get yourself all the more physically active and may have the option to appreciate somewhat more food, and some weeks you'll probably have slightly less activity and eat slightly less—there is no correct way to go about it. Attempt your best, refocus if you slip up, and never forget that you're in this for the long stretch, and consistency is all that matters.

Getting a charge out of the Foods You Like—in Moderation!

The last main advantage of cycling your carbohydrates is the best time—you can, in any case, appreciate the foods you like in moderation, and not feel limited. While you won't eat no-limit pizza and pasta regularly, when special occasions come up, or when you want to have fun, you can make these foods fit into your plan. Speaking carefully as far as fat loss is concerned, all that matters is the caloric deficiency. On a high-carb day, if you invest some of those carbs on a treat you appreciate, you can, in any case, get results.

Think about your daily calorie and macronutrient constrains as a bank account, and the amount of calories you ought to eat in a given day is how much cash you have available to spend. If it's a low-carb day and you just have 100 grams of total carbohydrates for the afternoon, you probably would prefer not to utilize 80 of them on a bag of candy or a bit of cake. You could do this, but then you'll have a lot harder time going carb-less the remainder of the day. However, if it's a high-carb day and you want to save some of them for dessert, that's acceptable. If it appears to be off-base that you can appreciate desserts in moderation and still get fit, simply remind yourself of the science. There are healthier decisions, sure, but as long as your total calories stay the same and allow you to stay under your caloric breaking point, there's no harm in getting a buzz out of something fun to a certain extent. You have to have self-control and be certain that one treat doesn't transform into the entire diet, but if you can learn to do that, you'll discover this diet considerably more sustainable. It's greatly improved to treat yourself now and then to eliminate all of the foods you appreciate until you reach your breaking point.

If having an occasional treat encourages you to stay on your plan, definitely use it. Life is meant to be enjoyed, after all, and this strategy for dieting can help you find that balance and happiness as you progress through your fat-loss venture.

CHAPTER THREE; HOW TO GET STARTED

Since you know the science behind carbohydrate cycling, the advantages, and the reasons it works so well, it's an ideal opportunity to dive into the practical side and start planning your new diet. You have to make sense of how to plan your high-and low-carb days, how many carbohydrates you ought to eat on those days, and how to plan for success. All of that will be shrouded in this chapter, which is your manual for assembling your first carbohydrate cycling plan.

Booking High-Carb and Low-Carb Days; The initial step is to choose when you will have high-carbohydrate days and when you will have low-carbohydrate days. There are a few ways to approach making sense of this, and several factors that will impact your choices. Personal inclination also has a job in making sense of this. Carbohydrate cycling is a hypothesis or practice, not an unbending, exacting diet plan. You can set up your plan to accommodate your life, your calendar, and your inclinations, and it will even now be powerful. The principal factor to consider is how many high-carb days you will have each week. Generally, this kind of plan works best when you have somewhere in the range of two and four high-carb days, two if you aren't extremely active and four if you are active, however, personal inclination and dieting history are also factors. If this is the initial time, you've tried to follow a diet plan, start with four high days, and gradually lower them. If you've been a diet meal for some time and are left with some difficult fat, you'll probably want to start with a few high-carb days.

Booking Your Days If You Aren't a Regular Exerciser; If you aren't doing a lot of physical exercises regularly, the days you decide for your high-carb days are a matter of personal inclination. It's ideal not to have them back-to-back, so you should attempt to spread them around the week. Think about your week after week calendar and social life. If you like to go out on the week's ends for food and beverages, you may want to have Friday or Saturday be a high-carb day, with different ones spread around the weekdays. Perhaps there's a night of the week where you join your work companions for a meal, in which case you may want that to be a high-carb day. Ultimately, it will come down to comfort and what works best for you. Planning

Your Days If You Are a Regular Exerciser; If you engage in physical exercise on week after week basis, you'll want to consider a couple of factors when planning your days. The physical exercise incorporates any activity you accomplish for 30 minutes or more with a moderate to high force level. If you go to the gym to lift weights, go for a run, or participate in a long climb or wellness class, those eventual exercise days. Extraordinary exercise exhausts glycogen and primes your body to absorb nutrients. Low-force activities, such as slow, restful walking—for example, walking around the mall—don't have the same impact.

If you follow an activity plan, at that point, you'll want to have your high-carb days on your most physically active days, as those days have the greatest requirement for fuel as glucose. You'll utilize glucose to exercise, and you'll use it to enable your body to recuperate, so it's a great time for higher carbohydrate intake. The planning of your food doesn't make a difference as some would claim, so don't go surging home to eat immediately after working out, but through the span of the day, you ought to have a higher intake. If your plan is three days of the seven days of weight training, which is a decent learner to-intermediate plan, make those your high-carb days. If you are trained on more than one occasion for every week, you can pick the third high-carb day. Not all exercise plans are three days, so if you are a following a four-, five-, or even six-day-out of each week program, or if you have a highly active activity, you'll have to do some reasoning. Consider which of those days are the most physically exhausting for you, or the hardest to recuperate from, and utilize those days as your high-carb days. If your resistance train, for example, generally, a lower-body workout is significantly more taxing than an arm or shoulder workout would be. Utilize those carbs to fuel your most exceptional activity.

Deciding Your Intake Levels Now; it's an ideal opportunity to make sense of exactly how much food you have to eat daily. It's important to realize that no calculation or estimation will ever be 100 percent accurate. Each individual is interesting, and this incorporates metabolic rates as well. These calculations may be accurate for some individuals but way excessively high or low for other people.

However, for a great many people, they are a decent starting point. It can all get somewhat precarious, so grab a pencil and paper and prepare to do some calculations. There are calculators online that work well, but here you'll learn how to do it manually.

Stage 1: Calculate Your Total Calories To start, you'll want to locate a total caloric intake goal for yourself. Again, this will simply be an estimate, but it may get you close. A decent rule is to take your total body weight and increase it by 12 if you are not very active and 14 if you are physically active regularly. To be physically active, you should either have a manual labor job or spend at least three to four days within the week doing a moderate-to high-force activity. As an example, a 180-pound male, increasing by 14 because he, as of late began an exercise program, would arrive at 2,520 calories (180 × 14 = 2,520). Again, this may be adjusted up or down contingent upon how he reacts, but it's a decent starting point.

Stage 2: Calculate Your Daily Protein Needs

Now that you have your total caloric intake, it's an ideal opportunity to break it down into macronutrients. Keep in mind, both a solitary gram of protein and a gram of carbohydrate has mainly 4 calories, whereas a gram of fat has 9 calories. It's a smart thought to aim for anywhere between 0.6 and 1 grams of protein for every pound of body weight, aiming for a higher-end if you are a regular exerciser. This may be the most important macronutrient and the one that doesn't change daily. For the original example, 1 gram for every pound would equal 180 grams each day, or 720 calories (180 × 4 =

720). As recently referenced, protein along with carbs is expected to recuperate, it fabricates muscle, keeps you full, and is extremely hard to digest. There is a factor called the TEF factor, or thermic impact of food. This alludes to the amount of energy it takes to break down and absorb the food you eat. That's correct—even the act of digesting your food consumes calories. Protein has the highest TEF factor, so you'll consume the most calories from digestion by eating protein. This, combined with the fact that it keeps you full, makes it invaluable for a tight eating routine.

Stage 3: Calculate Your Carbohydrate and Fat Need

At this point, how you distribute your remaining calories among carbohydrates and fat is largely a matter of personal inclination. It's a smart thought to have at least 20 percent of your total caloric intake originate from fat, as it's essential for many capacities in the body. There is no base for carbohydrate intake.

While calculating your macronutrient needs, never forget the total calorie transformations. 1-gram protein = 4 calories. 1-gram carbohydrate = 4 calories. 1-gram fat = 9 calories. It's extremely easy to overlook this and consider fat calories 4 as well, so be careful and double-check your numbers. How about we return to our example 180-pound male. If you recall, his total caloric needs were 2,520, with 720 being dedicated to protein each day. This leaves him with exactly 1,800 remaining calories to distribute as he sees best. If fat is to be kept at least 20 percent, some math can assist him with the rest. 20% of 2,520, the total calorie goal, is 504 total calories. To change over that to grams of fat, he'll separate this number by 9, as fat has 9 calories for each gram. This gives him 56 grams of fat at least each day. If you got lost there, take your total calories each day, duplicate it by 0.2, and then take whatever number you get, and separate it by 9.

While calculating your macronutrient needs, never forget the total calorie transformations. 1-gram protein = 4 calories. 1-gram carbohydrate = 4 calories. 1-gram fat = 9 calories. It's extremely easy to overlook this and consider fat calories 4 as well, so be careful and double-check your numbers. We should return to our example 180-pound male. If you recall, his total caloric needs were 2,520, with 720 being dedicated to protein each day. This leaves him with exactly 1,800 remaining calories to distribute as he sees best. If fat is to be kept at least 20 percent, some math can assist him with the rest. 20% of 2,520, the total calorie goal, is 504 total calories. To change that to grams of fat, he'll isolate this number by 9, as fat has 9 calories for every gram. This gives him 56 grams of fat at least each day. If you got lost, take your total calories each day, increase it by 0.2, and then take whatever number you get, and isolate it by 9.

He now has 180 grams of protein, 56 grams of fat, and the remaining calories are from carbohydrates. On a high-carb day, fat would stay low, around 56–60 grams, and the rest would be carbs. On a low-carb day, fat may increase to a fairly high amount. If total calories are 2,520, with the 180 protein and 56 fat established, that leaves 324 grams of carbohydrates for a high-carb day. On a low-carb day, if the carbohydrates were lowered to 200 grams, that would add an extra 55 grams of fat, bringing his daily total as high as 110. Keep in mind that total calories should stay the same, and protein should stay the same, so if you lower your carbs, you'll have to increase fat to reach your total caloric needs. If you got lost, here is a brisk recap of all the means:

- Multiply your body weight by 12–14 to get total caloric needs (12 for less active individuals, 14 for increasingly active individuals).

- Take 0.6–1 gram of protein for every pound of body weight; duplicate this by 4 to get total protein calories.

- Multiply the total number from stage 1 by 0.2 to get your base fat calories.

- Subtract your protein calories from your total calories, and the remaining calories can be part of carbohydrates and fat as you see fit.

Stage 4: Set Your Carb Numbers for High and Low Days

This boils down to personal inclination, and how your body reacts. Some individuals can have extremely high carb intakes and get exceptionally lean, and some need to keep their intake exceptionally low to lose fat. It will take some testing and trial and blunder to perceive how you react best. Take note of how you feel as far as energy, mood, and recuperation on low and high days, and adjust as required. To start with an estimation, aim for 1–1.5 grams of carbohydrate per pound of body weight on your high days and 0.5

grams per pound or less on your low days. On low days, contingent upon how low your carbs end up, you may be restricted to simply the trace carbs you'll discover in vegetables, and that's okay.

Meal Planning

Your Key to Success : The way to successfully hitting your goals each day is to plan. As long as you stay inside your caloric intake goals, you'll get results. If you can go much further and stay quite near your total protein, carb, and fat goals, you'll see far superior outcomes. However, if you don't plan, you'll have a hard time hitting your goals with any kind of accuracy, and no doubt, you'll wind up coming up short on a supplement or drawing near to your caloric breaking point before you are finished eating for the afternoon. The best activity is to invest some energy in creating a meal plan that allows you to stay inside your calories, and attempt to eat as near that plan as possible. It leads to being a lot of work in advance, but once you have a composed plan before you, following it is a lot easier than tracking as you go each day and adjusting on the fly. You'll want to think of a couple of sample days of eating, for high-and low-carb days. Along these lines, regardless of whether something comes up and you are unable to follow the plan exactly, you'll have an unpleasant idea of what your entire day should resemble, and you can plan. If you realize you'll have a lot of carbs for supper, you can take a gander at your plan and take those carbs out of different meals to save them.

Food Shopping and Grocery shopping ahead of time and preparing meals in advance are essential to your success, especially if you have a bustling calendar. There's nothing more awful than being extremely eager, not having the food you need around, and then having to pick between heading off to the store or requesting takeout. You'll require a lot of willpower in that situation, so it's ideal for planning simply. As you approach creating your meal plan, consider meals that are helpful to prepare and enjoyable for you. The recipes and sample meal plans in the back of this book will be useful in your planning. When you have your plan in place, it's easy to make a basic food item rundown of what you'll have to prepare your food, put in a couple of hours cooking it all, and put it away for it re-heating later. If you have an adaptable calendar without any duties, you may have the option to prepare your meals as new as you go, but there's nothing wrong with preparing all your food on the double and reheating as you need it. By planning, shopping, and investing some energy cooking, you can be certain that you have all the meals ready to go. You have a plan, and you have the food; all you need currently is simply the willpower and control to execute the plan and follow through.

Good and Bad Nutrient Combos; For the most part, you can technically eat any foods you want, at whatever point you want, and get results if the calories and macronutrients are correct. However, there is a major difference between something working and something being optimal. When planning your meals, there are a couple of supplement combinations to consider, and one, in particular, you want to avoid. Recalling carbohydrates trigger your body to release insulin, and insulin flips the switch that transforms your body into storage mode. If carbohydrates are in the meal, that meal will be absorbed and put away rapidly. As you may have the option to see, you must be careful with how you plan your meals if you want to streamline your advancement. By eating carbohydrates and proteins together, for example, after a workout, you can absorb and store the protein and carbs rapidly, which is something you want. Protein and fats together are a decent alternative when you want to stay full for some time. The two of them digest slowly, and the slow digestion will help give your body time to utilize them appropriately, rather than racing to store them in the most readily available place, which is your fat. The one combination you'll want to consider avoiding is carbohydrates and fat. If you have to consolidate them, it won't be the most terrible thing in the world—it won't cause you to gain instant weight or derail your advancement. However, for optimal performance, it's probably best to avoid this combination whenever the situation allows, or possibly keep fat low. If you raise your insulin, which makes your body want to store nutrients, and all you have floating around is glucose and fatty acids, chances are those that will go straight to your fat cells. Again, you can, in any case, get brings about the long haul, but this probably isn't a combination you won't regularly.

Booking "Cheat" Meals Straying off your plan because you didn't have self-control and ate way an excess of food isn't optimal. You can refocus, so there's no compelling reason to beat yourself up over it, but it won't help you accomplish your goals any faster. The beauty of this plan is that pretty much any food you want can be made to fit; you simply have to utilize moderation.

If you want to treat, or desserts, or a cut of pizza, it's more than okay to enjoy now and again; in fact, it's probably useful for your sanity, so you don't go crazy from opposing your favorite foods all the time. Simply make sure you plan. Reveal to yourself; you'll appreciate it without feeling regretful, make the most of your treatment, and get back on the program. If you don't have the self-control to stop with only a small segment, you may not want to go off plan excessively, but if you can handle it without eating everything in sight, pull out all the stops.

Tips and Tricks to Maximize Your Results

There are a couple of tricks and tips you can actualize that can help you reach your goals faster and make the entire procedure appear to be easier. These tips aren't anything magical, but as you become accustomed to following your plan, build up some reliable habits, and feel comfortable with what you are doing, these little can help take things to the next level.

Eat enough Carbohydrates Before and After Your Workouts; If you are active, it's a smart thought to eat a large part of your carbohydrates around your workout, anywhere from 30–50 percent, if not more. When you are pushing your body hard, you need legitimate fuel to perform at the highest level, and carbs will assist you with doing this. After an intense workout, your body will, in general, utilize any food you consume for recuperation and repair, so if you are working hard, any food you eat inside an hour or two of your workout will in all probability go to a helpful cause, rather than being put away as fat. If you want to have a high-carb meal, or plan a cheat meal, directly after an extreme quality training meeting is the ideal time.

Add Green Vegetables to Every Meal; Green stringy vegetables are a great way to add volume and fiber to your food without adding a ton of calories. Broccoli, spinach, kale, lettuce, and anything else green would be acceptable decisions. If you end up dropping your calories low to work off those last scarcely any difficult pounds, chances are you'll feel hungry for the day. Eating large parts of greens with your meals will go far toward keeping you full.

Drink Lots of Water within and Between Meals; Water is the essential thing you consume. It's also natural to feel like you are ravenous when your body is dehydrated and needs hydration. The two signals are fundamentally the same as, and hard to recognize. A decent principle is to drink a large glass of water with each meal, and taste water for the day between meals. If you detest drinking plain water, take a stab at utilizing new lemon, lime, or other organic product to add some flavor or attempt carbonated, flavored, zero-calorie waters.

CHAPTER FOUR ADVANCED CARB CYCLING STRATEGIES

At some point, you may run into staying focuses, or plateaus, while on your carb cycling venture. As you get leaner, you may have to utilize some fancy stunts to keep the outcomes coming. When you have mastered the basics of carb cycling, you can take several advanced advances to keep things moving and raise your outcomes to the following level. These strategies probably wouldn't be appropriate for someone who has quite recently started a diet but will work well if you've reached a certain degree of leanness and wind up stuck.

Adding Exercise

Carb cycling can be exceptionally successful all by itself. Regardless of your present health and wellness levels, cycling your carb intake can improve your body structure, mood, and an entire host of other health benefits. However, as you progress along with your adventure, you will probably run into plateaus. At the point when these situations happen, there are a couple of advanced strategies and tips you can actualize to get things going again.

Adding exercise to your daily life is the most productive way to lose body fat, increase a vast number of health indicators, for example, lowered circulatory strain and improved cholesterol levels, and avoid plateauing as you look for improved body synthesis. There are many ways to get active; it doesn't have to be constrained to setting off to the gym and working out or going for a run. Discover something you like, and work to make it a habit after some time.

All activities of human life consume calories. Eating, resting, digesting food, walking—it doesn't have to be an exercise for exercise if that isn't some tea. It's ideal for making a state of simply moving around additional for the day, as frequently as you can. Regardless of whether it's taking a walk around the area, taking the stairs instead of the escalator, or attempting another game, every piece adds up. Utilizing a pedometer or activity tracker can be a fun, motivating way to set daily goals for yourself and attempt to hit them. When starting an exercise program, you should start if you aren't utilized to regular physical activity. Start with a few times each week, for half an hour or something like that, and go from that point. You want to pace yourself; exercise should fit into your life, not make you worried and consumed. Keep in mind, you're in this for the long stretch, so there is no compelling reason to surge anything. Before embarking any exercise program, always check with your doctor to make sure you're cleared for that degree of physical activity.

Endurance Training versus Strength Training

So, you've chosen to get an exercise schedule; presently, it's an ideal opportunity to make sense of exactly what you plan on doing. Typically, with regards to working out, you'll likely observe endurance training and quality training as the two main sorts marketed for fat misfortune. While quality and endurance training have some overlap, overall, they are altogether different, and both have their place in a well-adjusted workout schedule.

Endurance training, or cardio, is generally remembered for a program to improve cardiovascular system health and consume calories. While you are active and your heart rate is elevated, you'll be consuming more calories than expected. Your cardiovascular system will be working hard, making it stronger and increasingly proficient over the long haul. After the activity, your body will gradually relax, re-entering to its normal state. During the activity itself, endurance training generally consumes more calories than quality training, which is why so many start running or walking to get in shape. With quality training, many variables become an integral factor, but the impacts are usually somewhat different from endurance training. Your heart rate will be elevated, for sure, but the amount of rest you take between your work-out sets and the total amount of work you do will have an impact. Quality training improves body organization by increasing lean bulk after some time, and with the best possible power, it has a strong positive impact on your hormones as well. It can also improve the act, lessen pain, and fortify your bones when done over an extensive period.

Starting an Endurance Training Program

Before embarking on any exercise program, always talk with your doctor. Exercise is distressing on your body, and if you have any conditions, including your heart or respiratory system, you may have specific cutoff points in place. When you have your doctor's clearance, it's an ideal opportunity to begin. Remember, the essential thing is to start slowly and develop your way after some time. Propelling yourself excessively hard, especially when simply starting another daily schedule, can be unpleasant. You have to work hard, but at a level that is appropriate for you. If you're simply starting, attempt to do 20–30 minutes two times every seven days of any activity. It tends to walk, riding your bicycle, going for a climb, a paddling machine at the gym—whatever you like. Rather than get into fancy heart-rate calculations or anything like that, simply aim to go at a pace that challenges you, but not to the point of being unable to wrap up. If you can hold a full conversation, it's probably excessively easy. However, if you are breathing so hard, you can't shape a sentence without getting discombobulated, that's excessive. Aim for somewhere in the center.

If you're further developed and are accustomed to going on long runs or running regularly, you'll have to discover ways to increase your power. Your body gets productive at things after some time, so if you started out practicing with 2-mile runs, which may appear to be inconceivably difficult from the get-go, eventually they will feel easy. You won't consume as many calories or see the same advantages. If you're an advanced endurance trainee, you'll either add more opportunities to your workouts or increase the force. Running slopes, utilizing interval training, or increasing the resistance on a bicycle or elliptical are all acceptable ways to increase your power. Always be certain you are challenging yourself appropriately.

Cycling Carbs Around Your Workouts

Planning your week with the goal that your high-carb days fall on your training days is extremely viable for getting the ideal outcomes. Deliberately practicing and pushing your body requires a lot more energy than essentially walking around and approaching your daily tasks. The body's favored fuel hotspot for exercise is glycogen, as it is the easiest to change over to useable energy. Glycogen originates from carbohydrates, which means that on workout days, there's a decent chance that the carbs you eat will be utilized to fuel your workout and/or help you re-spread from it. On days when you aren't training hard, you don't require as many carbs to work, which is why it is ideal to have high-carb days on your work-out days. if you want to take this above and beyond, it is worth taking a look at your supplement timing or eating plan. Ultimately, weight loss is constrained by total calories, so regardless of whether you don't follow a set eating plan, you can, in any case, observe great outcomes if you consume the correct amount of food each day. Timing your food intake, however, especially your carbohydrate intake, can improve both the quality of your workouts and your recuperation from them. It can help guarantee that the food you eat is utilized for maximum productivity. It's an advanced strategy that gives your body the greatest chance to utilize carbohydrates successfully, rather than putting them away as body fat. A decent way to try different things with this is to put about half of your total daily carb intake around your workout. If you've made sense of that, you will be consuming 200 grams on a workout day, take at least 100 of those grams and eat half previously and the other half after your workout. In addition to the fact that carbohydrates are utilized for fuel, but they are also important for recuperation. As you eat carbs, insulin spikes, which enables your body to drive nutrients into the muscles faster, bringing about improved recuperation. Stick with straightforward carbs that will be easy to digest, for example, natural products, rice, potatoes, and pasta. The exact planning isn't very important, but you should attempt to eat your pre-and post-workout carbs inside one to two hours before starting or closing your workout.

Breaking Through Fat-Loss Plateaus

If you've reached where you exercise regularly and have your high-carb days on your training days, and you're eating your carbs around your workouts, you may even now end up stalling out in your weight-misfortune venture. Here are a couple of further developed strategies you may want to consider if you are attempting to reach extremely low degrees of body fat and end up stalling or battling. They won't work for everybody, as individuals have different food inclinations and carbohydrate tolerances, but they merit attempting.

Is HIIT training, or interval training, beneficial?

HIIT training stands for high-power interval training. If you can't figure from the name, this kind of training is challenging, and should just be utilized by intermediate to advanced trainees. If you've been doing endurance training for some time and want to step up your game, intervals are a great way to do this. You could pick short intervals with higher forces, for example, fast runs for 10–20 seconds, or longer intervals at lower powers, something like a 1-minute run with a 1-minute walk for recuperation. Another example would be running at your top speed for 10 seconds, and then resting or walking slowly for 1 moment before repeating. As you improve your wellness levels after some time, you should hope to increase your week after week endurance training volume if you stall out and feel you need greater activity. If fat misfortune slows, you can either eat less food or consume more calories. If you want to consume more calories, you can simply make sense of how much cardio you are doing each week and do somewhat more. You can add 5–10 minutes to each meeting or add an extra cardio workout, but your goal should be to make a little progress through the span of the week. It's increasingly practical and easier to do somewhat more each day rather than attempt to do all of your cardio in one long session.

Strength Training Workouts

The number of strength-training workouts available can be overpowering. When starting, all you need is a well-adjusted full-body workout, which you can do a few times each week. Not far off, you can investigate different training parts and schedules, but until further notice, simply make sense of a decent standard that works for all the major muscle groups, and perform it as well as could be expected. Strength training doesn't always have to include weights or weight machines. You can get an extremely challenging training impact utilizing only your body weight and basic hardware available at home, for example, chairs and steps. If you like to be outside, you can work out at a park, beach, or playground. Joining a traditional Gym isn't necessary. It very well may be beneficial, depending upon your goals, but you can also get great results while never going to an exercise center. The following workouts can be performed a few times each week, and you should give yourself at least one day off in the middle of, to rest, and re-spread.

Sample Home Workouts

Joining a gym is great, but it very well may be costly or badly designed. If it's a possibility for you, it's a great tool to take advantage of. Still, if you are unable to join a gym in any capacity whatsoever, you can even now utilize exercise and strength training to drive yourself to the following level. Here are some basic bodyweight workouts you can do anywhere—if you have space to move, you can do these workouts.

There are two alternatives for the following workouts; A three-days-of the week beginner plan and a four-days-of the week intermediate plan. It's ideal to start with three days and go up from that point. With the fledgling plan, you'll have three full-body workouts to finish through the week; any days will work in as you don't do two back-to-back days. With the four-day plan, you'll have two chest area days and two lower-body days. You can do an upper and lower back-to-back, but you should take at least a day off to rest and recoup.

Full-Body Beginner's Workout

With this workout, you should finish all exercises, as fast as you can. Warm-up by doing bouncing jacks, a brisk walk or run, or anything else to get your heart moving for around 5 minutes before the workout. There is also an increasingly detailed warmup on the site, along with easier and harder renditions of each exercise. Attempt to rest for close to 15–20 seconds in the middle. At the finish of the workout, rest as long as 2 minutes until you feel recouped; at that point, repeat the entire circuit. Start by completing two rounds of the workout, and after multi-week, knock it up to three total rounds.

- Bodyweight Squats × 15
- Push-ups × 10
- Turn around Lunges × 10 for every leg.
- Plank × 30 seconds
- Superman × 15
- Glute Bridge × 15
- Bird Dog × 8 for each side

When you've reached where this feels easy, you can climb to the intermediate workouts. All of these workouts ought to be fairly fast once you learn the exercises, so if you want to add more, it wouldn't damage to take a walk, run, climb, or some other cardio activity after you are done.

Intermediate Workout

Much like the beginner's workout, you should finish all exercises as fast as you can. Move between exercises rapidly; at the end, rest until you feel recuperated; at that point, repeat the entire circuit. You ought to aim for three total rounds to start. If you want to make it all the more challenging, just decrease the amount of rest you take between adjusts. Make sure to visit the site for easier and harder variants of each exercise.

Chest area Workout

- Push-Ups × 25
- Superman × 20
- Side Plank × 30 seconds for every side
- Burpees × 10
- Reverse Crunch × 20
- Chair or Bench Dips × 15

Lower-Body Workout

- Bodyweight Squats × 25
- Side Lunges × 15 for every leg
- Glute Bridge × 25
- Split Squats × 15 for every leg
- Side Lying Hip Raises × 20 for each leg
- Reverse Lunges × 20 for each leg

When you've reached where the intermediate workouts feel easy, it may be an ideal opportunity to put resources into some exercise equipment or a gym enrollment. Certain muscle groups can be challenging to train with no equipment. If you find that you appreciate working out and want to accomplish increasingly, a gym maybe your best alternative. You can also discover training camps, work-outflanks, or many different wellness related group activities to appreciate that can blend things up and challenge you.

Cycling Carbs Around Your Workouts

Planning your week with the goal that your high-carb days fall on your training days is a compelling way to get the ideal outcomes. Intentionally practicing and pushing your body requires a lot more energy than essentially walking around and approaching your daily tasks. The body's favored fuel hotspot for exercise is glycogen, as it is the easiest to change over to useable energy. Glycogen originates from carbohydrates, which means that on workout days, there's a decent chance that the carbs you eat will be utilized to fuel your workout and/or help you re-spread from it. On days when you aren't training hard, you don't require as many carbs to work, which is the reason it is ideal to have high-carb days on your work-out days.

Staggered Carb Cycling

If you've steadily followed the basic template for some time, with high days and low days, it may be an ideal opportunity to start adding an intake somewhere in the center to vary significantly more. For example, you may have your high days set at 200 grams, and your low days set at 75 grams. If this has quit working, you may have the option to get things going again by really driving down those low-carb numbers and adding a center number. You may have 25-gram days, 100-gram days, and 200-gram days now, rather than necessarily high or low. The calendar could look something like this:

- Sunday: 25 grams carbs
- Monday: 25 grams carbs
- Tuesday: 25 grams carbs
- Wednesday: 100 grams carbs
- Thursday: 25 grams carbs
- Friday: 25 grams carbs
- Saturday: 200 grams carbs

As you can see, with a calendar this way, you'd have two squares of low-carb days followed by high-carb or re-feed. Varying your totals in such a way allows you to lower your overall caloric intake and have low carbohydrate intake for those couple of days. Remember that this is an advanced strategy, so there is no compelling reason to start with such low-carb days, except if you've been stuck for quite a while and can't find any other way to break your plateau. At the point when you utilize this technique, you should keep your protein and fat generally the same on all of the days. Keep in mind, by keeping your carbohydrate intake so low (at 25 grams), the greater part of the carbs you will eat will be trace carbs from fruits and vegetables; hence your calories will be meager. When you raise your carbs on your mid-and high-carb days, your caloric intake will increase, but this is completely fine. As long as you survive in a caloric deficiency for the entire week, you'll certainly get results.

The Weekly Depletion and Re-Feed

This advanced strategy puts all of your high carbohydrate intake toward the end of the week, or whatever two back to back days you pick, and lets you stay in a low-carb state all week. Many individuals have discovered success by staying trained with their diet during the week, at that point allowing themselves the end of the week to have an extremely controlled re-feed period. By having your high-carb days toward the end of the week, you can be additionally accommodating social occasions that include food and treat yourself a smidgen.

There may be physiological advantages to this strategy as well, not simply the mental break. As you get exceptionally lean, or if you've been dieting for an extended period, your metabolism can adjust, and weight loss can start to stall. If you've been working out hard and eating extremely confined calories, a sud-sanctum increase for a day or two can shock your body into fat-consuming mode again. If you've quite recently started a diet, you probably needn't bother with re-feed (or higher calorie) days, but if you've been crushing away at it for some time, it may be only the thing you need. If you pick this technique, you will profit most by lowering your total calories on your lower-carb days and raising your calories on your higher-carb, re-feed days. For example, if your daily average has been 2,000 calories, you could shift five low-carb days to 1,700 by lowering your carbs and fat, and your two re-feed days could be 2,750, with high carb intake. This will, in any case, make your daily total for the week average out to 2,000.

Carb Back-Loading

The last advanced strategy is carb back-loading. This will, in general assistance greatly with dietary adherence and may merit an attempt if you end up craving food and snacks late around evening time. The technique is straightforward—save all of your carbs for the day's end. It may appear to be outlandish, and you've probably read that eating after a certain season of the day makes you fat. There is no fact to this at all; all that matters is your total daily caloric intake. With carb back-loading, you make sure that your first meals and snacks are made of primarily lean proteins and some fats and vegetables. For your last meal of the day, you'll have all the remaining carbs. This could be a major bowl of rice or pasta, crackers, chips, or anything else you like and appreciate. You can head to sleep satisfied, you can lessen cravings, and if you love carbs, you give yourself something to anticipate at the finish of each day.

CHAPTER FIVE; THE MAINTENANCE PHASE

You should have no issues reaching your fat-misfortune goal if you can discover the willpower to stay with strong sustenance and exercise ace gram. It will take time, but if you can learn to appreciate the excursion, it won't be so bad. However, one thing frequently disregarded when talking about diets is what to do once you hit your goal. If you go directly back to your old habits, chances are you'll recover your old body. Many diets show dramatic when transformations, yet they don't mention to you what happens to those individuals once they attempt to return to a normal eating plan. You have to realize how to transition from your caloric deficiency phase to a normal, sustainable maintenance diet that allows you to keep and make the most of your new body. This chapter will show you how.

Do You Need to Carb Cycle Forever?

If you've reached your goal, you ought to have a supposition on carb cycling. You may love it or hate it, but ideally, it has helped you reach your goal without completely limiting or eliminating food sources. At the finish of a diet phase, you'll have to discover some way of eating that you will have the option to follow, that is tranquil, and that won't cause you to gain all your weight back inside those first few weeks. The beauty of carb cycling is that it doesn't necessarily mean you'll always track food, measuring things, and eating in a caloric shortage. They will have become your new dietary standard when you have learned the standards of carb cycling and utilized them to reach your goal. It's a style of eating you can follow as long as you wish with no negative symptoms. Cycling of your carbohydrate intake is probably perhaps the healthiest style of eating you can follow. Much after you work back up to where you are eating a lot more food again, you can, at present, reap all the health advantages of carb cycling, regardless of whether fat misfortune is a goal.

Keep in mind; carb cycling alludes to varying your carbohydrate intake on a day-to-day basis. It doesn't necessarily mean fat loss or weight gain; it's only a strategy. You can be carb cycling without actively attempting to get more fit; you can even carb cycle on a weight-gain plan. With some practice, you may have the option to reach where you can naturally eat without fanatically measuring everything and still maintain a healthy weight. This could mean eating more carbs around your workouts with less on-off days and mindfully watching your segments the remainder of the day without gauging all that you eat. Or then again, you may discover you appreciate the exactness of tracking food and having the ability to adjust your intake voluntarily to reach your weight goal. In any case, you can reach where you are eating the foods you appreciate regularly and still maintain your new body; it takes patience, self-control, and time.

Transitioning to a "Normal" Eating Style

Nobody wants to diet everlastingly, so it's important to return to a normal, or maintenance, level. Staying in a caloric shortage, long haul can have several negative symptoms. Your metabolism may slow down, thyroid activity can decrease, and the capacity and creation of different hormones can be negatively affected. These impacts are especially found in the individuals who have to bring their calories low to lose fat and stay like this for a sustained timeframe, for example, while preparing for a photoshoot or body challenge. Going back to a maintenance level in an effective way ought to be your first task after completing a diet. In addition to hormonal impacts, you also have a greater chance of passing important nutrients if you are in a caloric shortfall for quite a while. Regardless of whether all of your dietary decisions are natural, nutritious, entire food sources, you're despite everything going to eat less of them.

The Importance of Reverse Dieting

Turn around dieting is a term that alludes to increasing your caloric intake, slowly, over a given timeframe. Keep in mind; your body is brilliant. Similarly, as it adapts to running on decreased calories, which is why you may hit plateaus while dieting, your body can adjust to increased calories. By actualizing slow, strategic raises in your food intake, you can increase your food intake after some time without seeing a fast bounce back and weight gain. The goal with a turnaround dieting is to slowly increase your food intake, while limiting fat gain, not eliminating it. As an example, if you start a diet with a daily intake of 3,000 calories every day, shed 20 pounds, and end the diet eating 1,800 calories, you wouldn't have the option to hop directly back to 3,000 every day and keep all 20 pounds off. However, if you have the self-control to slowly and strategically increase your food after some time, you may have the option to return to 3,000 calories and keep 15 of those pounds off, in which case you're in a vastly improved place than when you started.

Metabolic capacity alludes to the number of calories your body runs on daily to maintain its present weight. If you eat 1,800 calories for each day and your weight doesn't change week to week, that's your maintenance level. Through hard work and careful planning, you may have the option to increase your body's metabolic capacity, allowing you to eat more while maintaining your present weight. You can also decrease your capacity through long haul caloric limitation or a sedentary lifestyle. Presently, suppose this same man instead takes the slow approach. After completing his diet, he increases his food from 1,900 to 1,950. He stays on this for up to 14 days, allows his body to body, and then increases to 2,100. He may gain a pound or two from extra water, but if he keeps the food constant and keeps on working out, his body will probably rebalance itself back out around his new weight of 175.

If he keeps adding small increases each seven to fourteen days, he will be slowly assembling his metabolic capacity or the amount of food he utilizes daily. Some weight gain may happen after some time, but it's entirely conceivable this man could increase his food intake back to 3,500 over a couple of months and still be inside five or so pounds of his new body weight. This approach takes patience and control, but it's the best alternative post-diet, except if you want to be in the dieting mindset perpetually, or gain all of your weight back. So many diets fail to address what to do once you hit your goal, presently, you know. There is no definite reason to discard the outcomes you've worked so hard for when you can learn to maintain them for the since quite a while ago run.

Carb Cycling for Maintenance and forever

As was quickly referenced previously, when you've reached your goal weight and have been there for some time, giving your body time to adjust and learn how to maintain its present degree of body fat, you can transition to a way of eating that doesn't require any special tracking. If you've reached your goal, you've probably learned how to adhere to a plan without straying excessively far and learned a bit of self-control as well. You can utilize these new skills to eat mindfully and maintain your new, lean body until the end.

Take a glance at what your eating habits were before you at any point began this diet, and be honest with yourself. If you just didn't know about how you ought to eat, you can probably shift into a maintenance mode fairly easily. However, if you realized what kind of foods you ought to eat and battled more with self-control or overeating, or couldn't avoid daily snacks and lousy nourishment, you may want to stay with tracking somewhat more and slowly ease into instinctual eating.

An ideal way to approach this is to make your meals comprising lean proteins, vegetables, and low to moderate amounts of fat. On days you will be engaging in resistance training or high-force exercise, eat some carbs previously, then after the fact. Rice, potatoes, organic product, or any other entire food carb source is acceptable here. On this, maybe on more than one occasion for each week, you ought to allow yourself to enjoy a bit. "Cheating" isn't the best word, as this can suggest an all-out eating meeting, but if you've been training hard and staying on track, having one meal with moderate bits of foods you appreciate won't hurt you. Here are some valuable and fast visual measurements for you. It's not necessary to fixate on the exact measurements, but it is useful to have the option to rapidly take a gander at food and estimate how much a serving is. When fabricating your meals, these are the rules that you should aim for.

- 1 is serving lean protein per meal—About the size of the palm of your hand.
- 1–2 handfuls of vegetables for each meal—Self-explanatory; generally, what you could gather up with a couple of hands.
- 1 small segment of fat with most meals—About the size of your thumb.

For entire eggs or fattier cuts of meat, no additional fat is required.

1 hold hand-measured serving of carbohydrates pre-and post-workout—Most of your meals will currently be extremely light on carbs. But the meals when your workout should each have a serving of carbs generally the size of your clench hand. If you discover you aren't recuperating well from workouts, go with two servings post-

workout. When you take a look at the sample meal plans at the finish of this book, you'll see workout days and rest days. Those days are set up in a way similar to what was simply portrayed: entire food decisions and carbohydrates around the workouts. You can eat whatever you like, as the plans are simply samples, but they are genuine examples of how you could structure your daily meals. If you are generally picking entire food sources and mindfully controlling your part measures, you shouldn't have an issue maintaining a healthy, lean body.

Intuitive Eating versus Carb Cycling

You can utilize general carb cycling to maintain your outcomes. For some individuals, this is easily sustainable, but others may not have the option to follow this. Some families regularly consume rice or beans as a staple fixing, or it may not be helpful to eliminate carbs. You may simply adore carbs and want them daily. If this is the case, you can, at present, maintain your outcomes and eat carbs daily; you'll simply have to be more careful. If you are carb cycling with entire foods and lean protein sources, just by their nature, you'll have a hard time overeating. It's hard, but not feasible, to gain fat eating lean meats or egg whites, vegetables, moderate fat, and restricted carbs. However, if you toss carbs in the mix, it gets much easier to gain fat, as they can pack a significant number of calories into your meals without keeping you full.

Ultimately what decides fat loss is total calories, no one macronutrient. Carb cycling holds your calories under tight restraints, but there is nothing magical about it. If you want to eat carbs daily, you can do this; you simply should be mindful of your total calories. When you are eating carbs with a meal, try to keep the fat on the lower end and still stick with your lean proteins. If you wind up gaining weight back, you may need to track again for possibly 14 days, see where you are overeating, and adjust accordingly. You can learn to instinctually eat for your body's needs, and make daily carbohydrate intake a regular part of your diet, but it may be somewhat harder.

Working in High-Carb Days Without Gaining Fat

All of this carb cycling and nourishment planning would be acceptable and well if life didn't disrupt everything. Social occasions will always come up, and you'll want to plan accordingly. Perhaps it's a wedding or party, and you know the snacks and beverages will be unending. Maybe it's a significant other's birthday or a vacation. It may very well be that you've been craving pizza all week and grab several slices and a lager on Friday after work. You can eat foods you appreciate without derailing your advancement. It just takes a tad of planning—and planning, if you will. Think about your week after week calories like a bank account. If you are eating your maintenance amount each day, you won't have a lot of extra to spare for the sake of entertainment purchases, or in this case, meals that you wouldn't normally eat. However, you can save your calories for that special occasion and still be completely fine. If you realize that you'll be feasting on Saturday night, rather than starving yourself all day to save calories and then overeating, you can eat somewhat less consistently. Maybe go for smaller bits, or forget that extra pastry or snack if you aren't ravenous and don't need it.

CHAPTER SIX; SAMPLE MEAL PLANS WITH RECIPES

This book incorporates more than 200 recipes for you to attempt. All sorts of foods are incorporated, separated into various categories. Additional information is incorporated with the recipes, but recipe results are probably going to vary from individual to per-child, so it's ideal for calculating that. If you need a place to discover nutritional information for food, even if you utilize the same fixings as given in the book, there are so many alternatives and brands for most food things that it's difficult to give nourishment information that will always be 100 percent accurate. Especially with entire foods that aren't mass-delivered the same way each time, serving sizes and sustenance substance will vary. However, you ought to have no issues with reading the recipes and concluding how to fit the ones you like into your day. The recipes are basic, without an excessive number of fixings, so a speedy read to perceive what goes into them should give you some information. There are also notes with each recipe that will assist you with night more. As a general standard, the majority of the recipes will incorporate a lean protein and low to moderate fat; if carbs are incorporated, that will be exceptionally clear. You can utilize recipes from any source you like and make them fit your sustenance plan, but the ones in this book will be a great starting point for you.

Sample Meal Plans

The meal plans in the book are meant to fill in as an example of how you could set up your day. An enlisted dietician or nutritionist did not plan them, so don't assume that by following them exactly as composed, you'll see dramatic outcomes; you, despite everything, need to make sure you utilize these recipes to hit you individualize caloric requirements. They are easy to prepare, tasty, and will assist you with reaching your goals, but they should be fit into your macronutrient needs. Everyone is different, so your plan ought to be worked around your life-style for best outcomes. The plans in this book simply show a general structure for various high-carb and low-carb days, with varying meal frequencies. You can utilize them as a sample of how a day may be set up. Regarding the matter of planning, you would profit by planning out a couple of days ahead of time to match your exact caloric needs. Having specific meals detailed, as you'll find in the sample plans, will let you see before the day even starts what your sustenance will resemble. Rather than planning each meal as you go, which is difficult and can be upsetting, it's best to prepare a plan and stick with it.

Question; Can't I simply eat different foods each day for a variety?

Ans; If you have much time or adaptability to eat whatever you want when you want, go for variety. Simply be mindful of this: it's easy to consume all of your carbs or fat earlier in the day than planned, leaving you with constrained decisions for your remaining meals. If you do stray from your plan, or want to substitute something else for a planned meal, you can rapidly glance over your meals for the afternoon, and stop mine was to make the change best.

If you have an extremely busy calendar or a family to take care of, planning your meals can make shopping and meal preparations a lot less difficult. You can pick snacks and snacks that are brisk and easy and prepare them in advance on a day if you have extra time.

Nutrient-Rich Vegetables

Prepare to eat a variety of nutrient-rich vegetables consistently. I'm talking about vegetables that are high in fiber and under 50 calories for every cup. You should eat at least 1 to 1.5 cups (cooked or raw) of nutrient-rich vegetables at 4 of your 6 daily meals. Keep in mind; you will eat your vegetables with your protein source before you eat any carbohydrates. Like protein, nutrient-rich, high-fiber vegetables assist you with feeling full. By eating your protein and vegetables first - and putting your fork down between nibbles - you will feel full faster, which keeps you from overeating.

Nutrient-rich vegetables approved for the Flexible Carb-Cycling Diet:

- Broccoli
- Salad (lettuce, romaine, and so on.); use non-fat dressing.
- Cabbage
- Green beans
- Spinach

- Zucchini
- Squash
- Red or green pepper
- Asparagus
- Carrots
- Tomatoes
- Cauliflower
- Mushrooms
- Artichoke hearts Carbohydrates

"Carb cycling" is a critical part of the Flexible Carb-Cycling Diet. This is the place you alternate between high-carbohydrate, low-carbohydrate, and no carbohydrate days. As I've referenced, you will expend carbs simply after eating your protein, vegetable, and natural product necessities for a given meal. It's simple:

- Day 1: High Carbs
- Day 2: Low Carbs
- Day 3: No Carbs
- Day 4: High Carbs
- Day 5: Low Carbs
- Day 6: No Carbs
- Day 7: High Carbs (and so on, following that cycle, for 30 days total).

Carbohydrates approved for Flexible Carb-Cycling Diet:

- Sweet potatoes or yams
- Brown rice
- Corn
- Peas
- Legumes (chickpeas, lima beans, lentils, dry beans)
- High-fiber cereals (All-Bran, Fiber One, Grape Nuts, Cracklin' Oat Bran, Shredded Wheat)
- Oats and oatmeal (not instant oatmeal)
- Black beans
- 100% wholegrain pasta (Eden, Hodgson Mill, Purity Foods)
- 100% whole grain bread (Pepperidge Farm, Nature's Path, Nature's Own, Earth Grains)

High-Carbohydrate Day

On this day, you will eat all the carbs you like until you reach completion. Again, you aren't stuffing yourself. You'll already have eaten your protein source, vegetables, and natural product, so you shouldn't be excessively hungry. Try not to feel bad for eating carbs. They assist you with softening fat and lose inches. Also, your body needs the calories from this energy source to keep the metabolism from easing back down and destroying your weight misfortune endeavors. As part of these high-carb meals, you should eat 1 bit of high-fiber organic product before the carbs. So, a meal on this day would resemble this:

High-fiber natural products approved for Flexible Carb-Cycling Diet:

- Raspberries
- Strawberries
- Blackberries
- Apple
- Pear
- Prunes
- Orange

Low-Carbohydrate Day

On this day, you will eat the same sorts of carbs as on the high-carbohydrate day, but you will intentionally limit your carb intake to just 2 of the 4-5 meals (which you don't have to do on the high-carb days). Again, devour your protein and vegetable servings first. At that point, eat 1 gram for every pound of your body weight of an "approved" carbohydrate hotspot for the afternoon. Partition this carbohydrate total by 2 and eat ½ of your total carbs at 2 of your 4-5 meals for the afternoon. This incorporates your bit of approved high-fiber organic product at each meal (to be eaten before the carbs). Below is an instance of how this works. A 205-pound man would devour 205 grams of "approved" carbs on "low-carb" days, with the goal that's 51.25 grams of carbs spread out more than 4 meals. Keep in mind; you eat carbs at just 4 of the 6 daily meals. The remaining

2 meals would be "no carbs," just protein and nutrient-rich vegetables.

Rules for No-Carb Days

It's important that you don't stray from the endorsed program. It was created along these lines for scientific reasons. Please DO NOT assume if you incorporate more "no-carb" days, you will show signs of improvement results. You won't. You are "cycling" these high, low, and zero carbohydrate days, so your body doesn't trigger its starvation reaction. Instead, it continues running at full productivity (meaning it consumes more calories). More isn't always better, and this is one of those instances. Trust me; if you follow the Flexible CarbCycling Diet exactly, you will see fantastic outcomes. So, don't get too suspended up on tracking calories. Earlier, we estimated your calories so you could use that value, as a rule, to make sure you are not eating close to anything or an extreme. If you put your fork down among chomps and carefully screen when you feel satisfied and not stuffed, you should never have to measure your caloric intake. Your low-carb day will be about equal to your caloric estimation. Your high-carb day will be somewhat higher, and your no-carb day a little lower. There is no compelling reason to measure your calories on your high-carb or no-carb days. Base your serving sizes on how full you feel, and not on what the calories or grams say.

Mostly follow the rules recorded above; in the request, they are recommended. If you need to have a reference point to work from, record how many grams of carbs and protein you eat for the initial days until you feel comfortable with how much food equals your protein and carbohydrate total for each day. Since we're on the subject of checking your eating, how about tracking your advancement, gauge yourself just once every 7 to 10 days. I recommend you weigh yourself in the first part of the day after a no-carb day. And think about taking different measurements, as well. Measure your hips, waist, legs, arms, and chest when the Flexible CarbCycling Diet.

Days Leading up to Your Event

In the last scarcely any days leading up to your occasion, you will change your carb cycle to a high, low, low, no-carb cycle. So if your occasion is on a Saturday, your timetable would resemble this:

- Tuesday; High carb
- Wednesday; Low carb
- Thursday; Low carb
- Friday; No carb
- Saturday; Day of the occasion (make it a low-carb day, if conceivable)

This will upgrade the Flexible Carb-Cycling Diet and have you looking lean and muscular on a big day.

CHAPTER SEVEN: RECIPES, BREAKFAST

1. Greek Egg Scramble

This tasty recipe is high in protein with low carbs and moderate fats. It is fast, easy to make, and a delectable meal. Adjust the fixings as required for personal inclination.

Ingredients

- Serves 1 2 large entire eggs
- 2 large egg whites
- 1 cup new spinach
- ¼ cup feta cheese
- 4 cup black olives (optional)
- ¼ teaspoon salt
- ⅛ teaspoon ground black pepper

High-Fat or Low-Fat?

Contingent upon your goals, you can adjust this recipe to have pretty much fat. Utilize entire eggs and full-fat cheese if you want progressively fat, or substitute in all egg whites and low-fat cheese if you want a lower-fat meal.

a. In a medium non-stick pan coated with cooking spray, add eggs and egg whites and set over medium heat.

b. Once eggs are partially cooked, about 3–5 minutes, add the remainder of the ingredient; mix until the eggs are not, at this point runny, and are cooked to your ideal consistency.

Per Serving

- Calories: 141
- Fat: 9g: 13g
- Sodium: 641mg
- Fiber: 0g
- Carbohydrates: 2g
- Sugar: 1g

2. Southwestern Omelet

This recipe packs a kick and is a great way to start your morning. Add as much hot sauce as you dare.

Ingredients

Serves; 1

- 1 entire large egg
- 2 large egg whites
- ¼ cup destroyed Mexican cheese mix
- ½ cup black beans washed and drained

- 1 tablespoon new cilantro
- ½ cup salsa, or to taste Dash hot sauce (optional)

Direction

a. Heat medium skillet coated with cooking spray or coconut oil over medium heat.

b. In a small bowl, blend egg and egg whites, utilizing a fork to break the yolk. Pour the blend in the pan and cook until it starts to set.

c. Add cheese, beans, and cilantro; cook 3 minutes, which overlaps over into omelet.

d. 4.Top cooked omelet with salsa and hot sauce if wanted.

Per Serving

- Calories: 389
- Fat: 20g
- Protein: 32g
- Sodium: 791mg
- Fiber: 7g
- Carbohydrates: 21g
- Sugar: 4g

3. Chocolate Banana Protein Pancakes

This tasty treat style breakfast will satisfy any sweet tooth while leaving you satisfied and full.

Ingredients; Serves 2

- ½ cup dry fast oats
- 1 medium banana, mashed
- 2 large egg whites
- 1 tablespoon chocolate chips Sugar or artificial sugar, to taste (optional)

The Power of Oats

Oats are a great replacement for flour and can be utilized in many recipes. For this and different recipes, you can utilize the oats as is, or mix them into powder utilizing a food processor or blender for better blending. This recipe can also be filled with a waffle maker.

Direction

a. In a medium bowl, join oats, banana, egg whites, and chocolate chips.
b. Pour even segments of the blend onto a frying pan or heated non-stick pan heated over medium heat.
c. When blend starts to air pocket and set, about 2 minutes for each side, flip over.
d. After expelled from the pan, pancake can be eaten as is or beaten with whatever you like.

Per Serving

- Calories: 192
- Fat: 3g
- Protein: 7g
- Sodium: 57mg
- Fiber: 4g
- Carbohydrates: 35g
- Sugar: 14g

4. Apple Cinnamon Oatmeal

This delectable fall treat is loaded with natural carbs and fiber and will keep you full and warm for quite a while. It can also be made in mass and reheated later.

Ingredients; Serves 2

- 4 cups of water
- 2 cups dry oats
- 1 large apple, diced, stripped if wanted
- 1 teaspoon cinnamon
- 2 tablespoons earthy colored sugar, or earthy colored sugar substitute

Direction

    a. In a large pan, heat water to the point of boiling.

    b. Add dry oats and cook according to headings on the package.

    c. After oats have cooked and thickened, lessen to a stew and mix in remaining fixings.

    d. 4.Cook 2–3 additional minutes, or until apple lumps have relaxed.

Per Serving

- Calories: 413
- Fat: 5g
- Protein: 11g
- Sodium: 23mg
- Fiber: 10g
- Carbohydrates: 83g
- Sugar: 25g

5. High-Protein French Toast

This take on classic French toast, is delectable and brimming with protein.

Ingredients; Serves 2

- 3 large egg whites, beaten
- 1 tablespoon each cinnamon and sugar
- ½ scoop vanilla protein powder (optional)

- 4 slices entire wheat or Ezekiel bread
- ¼ cup without sugar maple syrup

Protein Made Easy

This breakfast is a good way to get your carbs in the first part of the day, and it has a not too bad amount of protein. If you want to add more protein, you can blend protein powder into your cinnamon-sugar blend—it will work best with vanilla, cinnamon twirl, or unflavored protein powder.

Direction

a. Place whisk egg whites in a small bowl. Place cinnamon-sugar blend in a separate shallow bowl; blend in protein powder if wanted.

b. Dip slices of bread into egg whites, coating the two sides. At that point, plunge bread into a cinnamon-sugar blend.

c. Place coated bread onto a heated pan or skillet over medium heat. Cook 1–2 minutes each side.

d. Serve with without sugar maple syrup and any different fixings you like.

- Per Serving
- Calories: 216
- Fat: 2g
- Protein: 32g

- Sodium: 462mg
- Fiber: 1g
- Carbohydrates: 26g
- Sugar: 3g

6. Egg White Protein Bites

These low-carb, protein-packed powerhouses can be cooked in mass and refrigerated, and be ready to go whenever you need a breakfast on the run.

Ingredients. Serves; 4

- 2 cups egg whites
- 3 slices turkey bacon, chopped, uncooked
- ½ cup destroyed cheese, any sort
- ¼ teaspoon salt
- ⅛ teaspoon ground black pepper
- Pure Protein

These little snacks are loaded with complete protein and can have to such an extent or as minimal fat as you'd like with no carbs. You can utilize egg whites and turkey bacon, or blend in entire egg yolks or regular bacon if you want somewhat fatter and flavor with your meal.

Direction

a. Heat stove to 350°F. Spray a 12-cup biscuit pan with olive oil or any other cooking spray.
b. Fill each biscuit cup about ¾ full with egg whites.
c. Sprinkle bacon, cheese, salt, and pepper into the biscuit cups.
d. Bake 15 minutes, or until the egg whites have solidified.

Per Serving

- Calories: 142
- Fat: 6g
- Protein: 20g
- Sodium: 529mg
- Fiber: 0g
- Carbohydrates: 1g
- Sugar: 1g

7. Power Wrap

This power wrap is loaded with all of your macronutrients—protein, carbs, and fat. It's a great alternative when you realize you won't get food for some time, or essentially want a satisfying higher-calorie breakfast.

Ingredients

- 1 2 large entire eggs
- ½ medium avocado, stripped, pitted, and cut

- ¼ cup destroyed cheese, any benevolent 1 strip cooked turkey bacon
- 1 (8") entire wheat tortilla

Why Avocado?

Avocados are an awesome wellspring of potassium and monounsaturated fat, a great kind. They can be utilized for substantially more than guacamole, as this recipe shows. If you want less fat, you can always avoid avocado.

Direction

a. In a medium pan, low the gas, scramble eggs to your ideal consistency.
b. Place eggs, avocado slices, cheese, and bacon into the tortilla and move it up.

Per Serving

- Calories: 446
- Fat: 29g
- Protein: 25g
- Sodium: 732mg
- Fiber: 3g
- Carbohydrates: 20g
- Sugar: 2g

8. Two-Minute Chocolate Strawberry Protein Bowl

This speedy and easy breakfast is brimming with protein, micronutrients from the organic product, and antioxidants. This is a very filling and easy breakfast for those with a bustling calendar.

Ingredients

Serves; 1

- 1 cup non-fat pure Greek yogurt
- 1 cup new or solidified cut strawberries
- 1–2 tablespoons dark chocolate lumps
- 2 tablespoons sans sugar chocolate syrup 1 scoop chocolate whey protein powder (optional)

What Is the Best Greek Yogurt?

Nowadays, there are so many alternatives for Greek yogurt. Your most logical option is to go with something unflavored, to avoid extra sugar and carbs.

Direction

You can utilize low-fat or full-fat contingent upon your inclination. In a medium bowl, join all ingredients and blend. The whey protein is optional, but an easy way to get an extra 20–25 grams of protein into your daily intake.

Per Serving

- Calories: 434
- Fat: 11g
- Protein: 40g
- Sodium: 215mg
- Fiber: 9g
- Carbohydrates: 46g
- Sugar: 35g

9. Protein Scramble Bowl

This recipe is a decent way to get healthy fats, total proteins, and an entire bundle of micronutrients.

Ingredients

- 1 2 large entire eggs
- 2 2 large egg whites
- 3 1 cup fajita vegetable blend (solidified or newly cut)
- 4 1 turkey sausage connect, cooked
- 5 ¼ cup destroyed sharp Cheddar
- 6 ¼ teaspoon garlic salt

Direction

a. Combine all ingredients to an average skillet over medium heat.
b. Scramble blend until it reaches your ideal consistency.

Per Serving

- Calories: 469
- Fat: 26g
- Protein: 44g
- Sodium: 1,439mg
- Fiber: 4g

- Carbohydrates: 17g
- Sugar: 1g

10. Low-Calorie Bacon, Egg, and Cheese

This breakfast classic can easily be made utilizing exceptionally low-calorie ingredients without sacrificing any taste. This breakfast is brisk, easy, and sure to please.

Ingredients

Serves; 1

- 1 entire grain English biscuit 1 large entire egg
- ¼ teaspoon salt
- ⅛ teaspoon ground black pepper
- 1 cut cooked turkey bacon
- 1 cut without fat cheese

Boost Your Fiber with Breakfast

It is important to remember fiber for your diet, as it helps keep your digestive system working. The best way to fulfill this is to look for high-fiber bread and English biscuits, as you can usually discover these with extra fiber to keep you feeling full and keep your body healthy.

Direction

a. 1.Slice English biscuit and place in a toaster.

b. 2. While it is toasting, cook an egg in a medium skillet over medium heat to your ideal consistency (over easy, over medium, and so forth.) Add salt and pepper.

c. 3. Place egg, cooked bacon strip, and cheese in toasted biscuit and appreciate.

Per Serving

- Calories: 308
- Fat: 13g
- Protein: 24g
- Sodium: 1,019mg
- Fiber: 1g
- Carbohydrates: 24g
- Sugar: 2g

11. Vanilla Raspberry Protein Fluff

This flavorful treat could almost be viewed as a pastry, but it is a very fulfilling breakfast that will keep you full and empowered for the duration of the morning.

Ingredients

Serves; 2

- ½ cup solidified raspberries
- 2 scoops vanilla protein powder (casein is suggested; whey can also work)

- ¼ cup unsweetened vanilla almond milk 1 (3.5-gram) packet stevia, or your sugar of decision

What Does Fluff Refer To?

By blending all the recipe in a bowl, you already have a satisfying, filling treat. However, if you have a blender available, handling this blend for 5–10 minutes can double or triple the volume, making this taste like fruity whipped cream.

Direction

- Slightly thaw berries, so they are as yet chilly, but delicate.
- Add all recipes to a small bowl and mix; you ought to have a thick, pudding-like surface.
- Eat as is, or blend in a power blender 5–10 minutes until blend cushions up.

Per Serving

- Calories: 186
- Fat: 1g Protein: 26g
- Sodium: 56mg
- Fiber: 3g
- Carbohydrates: 19g
- Sugar: 16g

12. Berries and Cream Parfait

A fun and sweet breakfast, ideal for a relaxing day. You can pick high-or low-fat ingredients and make this fit whatever your caloric goals are for the meal.

Ingredients

Serves; 2

- 1 cup vanilla Greek yogurt
- ½ cup new blueberries
- ½ cup new blackberries
- ½ cup new raspberries
- ½ cup without fat whipped cream
- ½ cup granola or high-fiber cereal

Micronutrient Powerhouse

Berries are exceptionally wealthy in antioxidants, which help your body to expel damaging free radicals caused by pressure or exercise. Utilize any berries you'd like in this recipe, picking a variety of hues to get a more extensive choice of nutrients.

Direction

In a parfait glass or bowl, create layers with your ingredients for a visually pleasing meal. Rather, you can combine all the ingredients in a medium bowl and enjoy it.

- Per Serving
- Calories: 305
- Fat: 9g
- Protein: 12g
- Sodium: 89mg
- Fiber: 8g
- Carbohydrates: 46g
- Sugar: 30g

12. Spinach, Red Onion, and Mushroom Frittata

A delicious combination of iron-rich spinach and antioxidant-packed red onion and mushrooms, this frittata conveys lots of tasty sustenance.

Ingredients

Serves 6

- 6 large entire eggs
- 2 tablespoons water, partitioned
- ½ cup cut or diced red onion
- 1 cup cut mushrooms
- 1 cup new spinach
- 1 teaspoon all-natural sea salt

- 1 teaspoon cracked black pepper

Bone Benefits of Spinach

While spinach has, for quite some time, been perceived as a nutritious green for its high substance of iron and complex carbohydrates, the vitamin K substance of this superfood is far increasingly amazing. With each cup of cooked spinach comes more than 181 percent of the daily recommendation for vitamin K, which has the primary job of forestalling bone misfortune and advancing bone strength. By restraining osteoclasts' activity (cells that act to deteriorate bone) and giving sustenance to osteoblasts (cells that construct bone and bolster their structure), spinach's heavy portion of vitamin K is an essential part of any diet needing bone-supporting advantages.

Direction

a) Preheat oven to 350°F.
b) In a blending bowl, ultimately consolidate the eggs and 1 tablespoon of water.
c) Preheat a large, ovenproof skillet above medium heat, and spray with non- stick spray.
d) Add 1 tablespoon of water and the red onion to the skillet and sauté until somewhat mollified about 2 minutes.
e) 5Add the mushrooms and the skillet, then sauté for 2 minutes.
f) 6Add spinach to the skillet and sauté for 1 moment before adding the egg blend.

g) Place the whole skillet into the stove and bake for 20 minutes, or until firm to contact.

h) Season with salt and pepper.

Per Serving

- Calories: 82
- Fat: 5g
- Protein: 7g
- Sodium: 468mg
- Fiber: 0.5g
- Carbohydrates: 2g
- Sugar: 1g

13. Huevos Rancheros

Packed with clean ingredients that all give quality nourishment, these Huevos Rancheros are a healthier variant that you can actually like eating.

Ingredients

Serves 4

- (8") whole wheat tortillas
- 8 large whole eggs
- 1 tablespoon water
- 2 cups Fresh Salsa (see sidebar)

- 2 tablespoons chopped new cilantro

Fresh Salsa

- In a large bowl, join 2 large beefsteak tomatoes,
- chopped; 2 medium avocados, stripped and chopped;
- 2 large red onion, stripped and chopped;
- ½ large red ringer pepper, chopped;
- ½ small jalapeño, chopped and seed-ed;
- 2 cloves garlic, squashed;
- ¼ cup newly pressed lime juice;
- 3 tablespoons chopped cilantro;
- 1 teaspoon bean stew powder; and
- ¼ cup olive oil. Cover and refrigerate 2–12 hours before serving.

Direction

a. In a large skillet prepared with non-stick spray over average heat, warm tortillas individually, about 1–2 minutes. Rapidly wrap with tinfoil to keep warm until use.

b. Spray skillet with progressively non-stick spray and add the eggs carefully, not breaking the yolks—Cook up to 3 minutes, or until it turns out to be white.

c. Add 1 tablespoon of water and spread. Keep cooking for 3–5 minutes, until wanted doneness is achieved.

d. Lay 1 tortilla on each of four plates; top with 2 eggs each.

e. 5.Return saucepan to heat and add salsa to skillet, always blending for 1–2 minutes or until heated through.

f. Top each tortilla's eggs with ½ cup of warmed salsa, and garnish with chopped cilantro.

Per Serving

- Calories: 271
- Fat: 12g
- Protein: 17g
- Sodium: 1,108mg
- Fiber: 3g
- Carbohydrates: 24g
- Sugar: 5g

14. Basic Sweet Potato Pancakes

Sweet, fleecy, and packed with clean, complex carbohydrates, this brilliantly shaded breakfast alternative is fast, easy, nutritious, and heavenly!

Ingredients

Serves 10

- 1 cup yam purée
- 1 cup low-fat plain Greek yogurt
- 1 cup unsweetened applesauce

- 2 large egg whites
- 2 large entire eggs
- 2 teaspoons vanilla extract
- 2 tablespoons Sucanat
- ¼ cup 100% entire wheat flour
- 1 teaspoon baking powder
- 1 teaspoon pumpkin pie zest
- 1 teaspoon cinnamon
- 2 tablespoons agave nectar

Direction

a. Coat a large non-stick saucepan with olive oil cooking spray and place over medium heat.

b. In a large bowl, consolidate all ingredients except the agave nectar and blend well.

c. Scoop the batter onto the preheated skillet, utilizing approximately ½ cup of batter per pancake.

d. Cook 2 to 3 minutes on both sides or until brilliant earthy colored. Expel from heat, plate, and shower all pancakes with the agave nectar.

Per Serving

- Calories: 78
- Fat: 1g
- Protein: 7g

- Sodium: 52mg
- Fiber: 1g
- Carbohydrates: 13g
- Sugar: 6g

15. Clean Protein Power Bars

Rather than choosing a locally acquired variant, attempt these tasty homemade power bars for breakfast. Not exclusively are they the ideal arrangement of muscle-advancing protein, there's the added advantage of an explosion of heavenly flavor in each nibble.

Ingredients

Serves 9

- 4 cups moved oats
- ¼ cup entire wheat flour
- ¼ cup ground flaxseed
- 2 large entire eggs
- 1 cup all-natural almond butter
- ½ cup plain or vanilla almond milk or soymilk
- 2 tablespoons chopped or fragmented almonds

Anti-inflammatory Benefits of Flaxseed

With regards to the great wellsprings of omega-3 fatty acids, the vast majority consider fish being the best supplier. Flaxseed is one of the lesser-known foods that packs enough of this essential acid to diminish inflammation and debilitating conditions that outcome greatly. In only 2 table-spoons of flaxseeds, more than 130 percent of the suggested daily intake for omega-3s is given. Asthma, osteoporosis, osteoarthritis, rheumatoid arthritis, and even migraines can all be improved with the regular incorporation of flavorful flaxseeds in any diet.

Direction

a. Spray a 9" × 9" glass pan with olive oil spray and preheat oven to 350°F.

b. In a large bowl, join oats, flour, flaxseed, eggs, almond butter, and almond or soymilk, and mix thoroughly.

c. Pour the blend into the prepared pan and spread uniformly. Top with chopped or fragmented almonds, pressing them gently into the highest point of the mix.

d. Bake for 25–35 minutes, or until firm.

e. Allow to sit for 1 hour before cutting into 9 equal squares.

Per Serving

- Calories: 382

- Fat: 26g
- Protein: 8g
- Sodium: 27mg
- Fiber: 4.5g
- Carbohydrates: 28g
- Sugar: 1g

16. Homemade Scallion Hash Brown Cakes

Traditional fat-laden recipes of this breakfast favorite get cleaned up in this as good as ever form by utilizing heart-healthy olive oil and new ingredients that give complex carbohydrates and antioxidants in each firm cake.

Ingredients

Serves 6

- 3 Idaho potatoes, stripped and destroyed
- 1 cup chopped scallions 1 entire large egg
- 2 tablespoons 100% whole wheat flour
- 1 teaspoon garlic powder
- 1 tablespoon extra-virgin olive oil
- 1 teaspoon all-natural sea salt

- ½ teaspoon cracked black pepper

Better Your Brain Functioning with Better Potatoes

Because potatoes have a bad reputation as an unhealthy starchy carbohydrate, it's essential to clarify the advantages of including clean potato recipes in your diet. With a solitary potato giving a slam ping 20 percent of your daily suggested vitamin B6 intake, a meal including a baked, sautéed, steamed, or mashed potato contributes to the health of your brain's procedures by concentrating on the most intricate of all its parts: the cell. Advancing cell creation, cell regeneration and repair, and cell working and communication, potatoes' arrangement of B6 can help support your brain work.

Direction

a. Spray a big saucepan with olive oil and place over medium heat.

b. In a large blending bowl, consolidate destroyed potatoes, scallions, egg, flour, and garlic powder.

c. Form potato blend into 6 even servings, and form into thick patties.

d. Heat the olive oil in the skillet for 1 moment and twirl to equally coat.

e. Add patties to the skillet, three at a period, cooking 5–7 minutes for each side or until brilliant earthy colored and cooked through—season with salt and pepper.

Per Serving

- Calories: 131
- Fat: 3g
- Protein: 4g
- Sodium: 412mg
- Fiber: 2g
- Carbohydrates: 22g
- Sugar: 1.5g

CHAPTER EIGHT; LUNCH

17. Shrimp Stir-Fry

Cooking a major pan-fried food at the start of the week is a really easy way to have snacks ready for the week. You can store the prepared food in containers in the refrigerator and reheat over the oven or in the microwave at whatever point you need a fast meal.

Ingredients

Serves 2

- 1 (16-ounce) bag solidified sautéed food vegetables
- 1 tablespoon olive oil
- 6 ounces shrimp, thawed
- ¼ teaspoon minced garlic
- ¼ teaspoon sea salt

Carb It Up

You can eat this sautéed food as is, for a protein and vegetable meal that packs a lot of nutrients. If you want to add some carbs, you can present with rice, quinoa, pasta, or any other carb of decision. It's great as is, but also a decent addition to a bowl of rice if you want a snappy post-workout meal.

Direction

a. In a large pan, set a medium heat, cook vegetables with olive oil.

b. Add the remainder of the ingredients, and cook until shrimp are thoroughly cooked (they will turn opaque and pinkish), usually around 5 minutes.

Per Serving

- Calories: 240
- Fat: 9g
- Protein: 22g
- Sodium: 486mg
- Fiber: 6g
- Carbohydrates: 20g
- Sugar: 0g

18. Slow-Cooked Chicken

This is the most versatile way to cook your chicken. It stays delicate and soggy, and it goes with anything. You can make it into a sandwich, add it to a salad or rice, or simply eat it.

Ingredients

Serves 4

- 1-pound boneless, skinless chicken breast
- 1 (16-ounce) box low-sodium chicken stock
- 1 medium white onion, stripped and cut
- ¼ teaspoon garlic salt
- ⅛ teaspoon ground black pepper

The Tastiest Chicken

Slow cooking may very well be the ideal way to cook chicken. Baking and barbecuing are fine, but the chicken has a propensity to dry out when cooked with these strategies. After slow-cooking, your chicken will fall apart and shred easily and retain a lot of its dampness. The flavor is full but not overpowering, so you can add it to different dishes or sauces without negatively impacting the flavor of the meal.

Direction

a. Trim and clean chicken and place in the base of a slow cooker.

b. Pour in enough chicken stock allow it to cover the highest point of the breast.

c. Add onion and seasonings to the slow cooker.

d. Cover then reduce the cooker and cook on low setting 4 hours until chicken is done.

  e. Remove and shred with a fork. It tends to be eaten immediately or saved for later use.

Per Serving

- Calories: 199
- Fat: 5g
- Protein: 27g
- Sodium: 914mg
- Fiber: 0g
- Carbohydrates: 10g
- Sugar: 1g

19. Turkey Burgers

Turkey burgers are fast to prepare and extremely easy to transport. Eat them cold, reheat them, or break them up and add them to another meal.

Ingredients

Serves 4

- 1-pound ground turkey
- ¼ teaspoon salt

- ⅛ teaspoon ground black pepper

- ¼ cup bread pieces

Ground Turkey—Your Secret Weapon

It tends to be hard to reach your protein goal. A decent trick is to just cook a lot of ground turkey in a pan with minimal seasoning. You can store this, and then add it to pasta, eggs, burritos, or any other dish that needs a protein help, as it's a versatile addition without an overpowering flavor.

Direction

a. Combine all ingredients in a large bowl.
b. Mix well; at that point, utilize your hands to shape into 4 even burger patties.
c. Grill or cook in a skillet until burgers are cooked all the way through, about 3–4 minutes for every side.

Per Serving

- Calories: 194

- Fat: 10g

- Protein: 20g

- Sodium: 302mg

- Fiber: 0g

- Carbohydrates: 5g

- Sugar: 0g

20. Spaghetti Squash Crab Blend

This dish is easy to make, tasty, and supplies some filling carbohydrates, so you have the energy for your day.

Ingredients

Serves 2

- 1 medium spaghetti squash
- 1 (6-ounce) package imitation crab meat (or 1 (6-ounce) can real lump crab meat)
- ½ teaspoon Old Bay seasoning,
- ¼ teaspoon salt
- ⅛ teaspoon ground black pepper

Direction

a. Preheat oven to 400°F.

b. Carefully cut squash down the middle the long way and place cut side up on a baking sheet. Bake until squash is delicate, about 30–45 minutes relying upon the size of the squash.

c. Peel squash away from the skin with a fork and place strands in a medium bowl.

d. 4. Add the crab meat and seasonings and blend well.

Per Serving

- Calories: 82
- Fat: 1g
- Protein: 15g
- Sodium: 521mg
- Fiber: 1g
- Carbohydrates: 3g
- Sugar: 2g

21. Spinach, Feta, and Pesto Chicken Quesadillas

Quesadillas are exceptionally speedy to put together, especially if you use pre-made ingredients. You can cook and eat them new, or cook them ahead of time and reheat them later if you have to take them somewhere.

Ingredients

Serves 1

- 2 tablespoons pesto spread
- 1 (8") entire grain tortilla or flatbread
- 4 ounces destroyed chicken (see Slow-Cooked Chicken recipe in this chapter)

- ½ cup new baby spinach
- ¼ cup feta cheese

Homemade Pesto

Homemade pesto will set this recipe off if you have some free time and want to flavor things up. We have a lot of recipes out there to attempt, but for a straightforward one, take new basil with a little minced garlic and mix in blender or food processor with a little olive oil. Adjust segments to taste.

Direction

a. Spread pesto all over the tortilla and fill one half of tortilla with the chicken, spinach, and cheese.

b. Fold tortilla into two and cook in a medium non-stick pan over medium heat.

c. Flip once the base is brilliant earthy colored, earthy colored the opposite side, at that point serve and appreciate.

Per Serving

- Calories: 645
- Fat: 26g Protein: 41g
- Sodium: 1,404mg
- Fiber: 4g

- Carbohydrates: 57g

- Sugar: 4g

22. Low-Fat Chicken Bacon Ranch Sandwich

Here is an excellent alternative to a chicken bacon ranch sandwich that is low-fat, tasty, and packed with protein and high carbohydrates.

Ingredients

Serves 1

- 2 slices entire grain bread

- 3 ounces flame-broiled chicken breast

- 2 slices cooked turkey bacon

- 2 tablespoons sans fat ranch dressing

The Best Bread?

As far as unadulterated calories, there is undoubtedly not an immense variety among various bread manufacturers. You'll likely locate that most slices range from 80–140 calories. For maximum health, however, a grew, whole grain bread will be brimming with fiber and beneficial nutrients.

Direction

a. Toast bread.

b. On one cut bread, layer chicken breast then bacon. Spread ranch dressing throughout the second cut of bread and utilize that piece to top the other. Serve.

Per Serving

- Calories: 442
- Fat: 390g
- Protein: 37g
- Sodium: 1,438mg
- Fiber: 2g
- Carbohydrates: 38g
- Sugar: 2g

23. Sirloin Chopped Salad

A flavorful low-carb salad choice that's somewhat more intriguing than your standard flame-broiled chicken salad and contains a variety of healthy fats to keep you full.

Ingredients

Serves 1

- 4 ounces cooked sirloin, cut
- 2 cups blended greens

- ¼ cup blue cheese disintegrates

- 1 tablespoon chopped nuts, any sort

- 2 tablespoons balsamic vinaigrette, or dressing of decision

Direction

Place sirloin, greens, cheese, and nuts in a large bowl and blend to join. Top with balsamic vinaigrette or a dressing of your decision.

Per Serving

- Calories: 586

- Fat: 38g

- Protein: 46g

- Sodium: 573mg

- Fiber: 6g

- Carbohydrates: 11g

- Sugar: 3g

24. Southwestern Fajitas

Fajitas are a truly adaptable meal. When this filing is cooked and prepared it very well may be reheated and eaten alone, or presented with tortillas and rice for extra carbs. Serve these fajitas with destroyed Mexican cheese and low-fat sharp cream if desired.

Ingredients

Serves 2

- 6 ounces boneless, skinless chicken breast, cut into strips
- 1 teaspoon red pepper flakes
- 1 teaspoon fajita or taco seasoning
- 1 (16-ounce) bag blended fajita vegetables Dash hot sauce

Direction

a. In a medium skillet with low heat, cook the chicken, seasoned with red pepper and fajita seasoning up to 8–10 minutes; until chicken is not, pink.
b. Once cooked, expel, and put in a safe spot.
c. In the same skillet, add vegetables and cook 5 minutes or until soft.

When vegetables are cooked, add the chicken back to the pan, add a dash of hot sauce or more to taste, and cook until heated through.

Per Serving

- Calories: 186
- Fat: 3g Protein: 23g
- Sodium: 226mg Fiber: 6g
- Carbohydrates: 19g
- Sugar: 0g

25. Tuna Salad

This classic lunch can be filled in as a sandwich, eaten with crackers, or eaten plain. It rushes to make in large batches so you can have extra meals if you are in a surge and don't have time to cook, and it's easy to transport if you need lunch in a hurry.

Ingredients

Serves 1

- 1 (5-ounce) can tuna
- 2 tablespoons low-fat mayonnaise
- 1–2 tablespoons finely chopped celery
- Dash lemon juice
- ¼ teaspoon salt
- ⅛ teaspoon ground black pepper

Does Canned Tuna Have Healthy Fats?

You may see advertising on tuna cans that it is high in omega-3s, a good fat. While this is valid for the whole tuna, it isn't always evident with canned tuna. Take a look at the nourishment label and get tuna with higher fat if you want the omega-3s. If you advertise high omega-3s, but a serving has only 0.5 grams of fat, you aren't getting many omegas. Search for albacore tuna, rather than light tuna in water, if you want the omega-3s.

Direction

Tuna packed in oil will usually simply have higher fat because of the oil itself. Transfer all ingredients in a small dish and blend to consolidate. Chill until ready to serve.

Per Serving

- Calories: 264
- Fat: 11g
- Protein: 36g
- Sodium: 1,238mg

- Fiber: 0g
- Carbohydrates: 3g
- Sugar: 2g

26. Chicken Nachos

This delicious and protein-packed snack is a great way to satisfy cravings and get a well-adjusted meal containing protein, carbs, and fat.

Ingredients

Serves 1

- 1 serving (according to package) whole-grain tortilla chips 3 ounces destroyed cooked chicken
- ¼ cup low-fat destroyed cheese, any sort
- ½ cup salsa
- ¼ cup low-fat acrid cream

Direction

a. Heat oven to 375°F.
b. Spread chips on baking pan secured with aluminum foil, and top with cooked chicken and cheese.
c. Cook 12–15 minutes. Evacuate and present with salsa and acrid cream.

Per Serving

- Calories: 521
- Fat: 19g
- Protein: 39g
- Sodium: 1,379mg
- Fiber: 5g

- Carbohydrates: 36g
- Sugar: 7g

27. Healthy Fried Rice

While not a traditional singed rice dish, this Asian meal is speedy and enjoyable. It may be eaten alone or filled in as a side with another dish. This is a superb wellspring of speedy digesting carbs for pre-or post-workout.

Ingredients

Serves 2

- ½ cup egg whites
- 1 cup cooked rice
- ½ cup raw blended small vegetables (peas, carrots)
- ½ teaspoon soy sauce

What kind of Rice is the Healthiest

It doesn't make a difference what kind of rice you use. White rice, earthy colored rice, jasmine rice, and wild rice all have fundamentally the same as nutritional substances. You may have heard that earthy colored rice is healthier, but the main real difference is the speed of absorption. Earthy colored rice absorbs all the more slowly, but some individuals have issues digesting it, so it's a personal preference.

Direction

a. In an average skillet, lower the heat, cook egg whites to your desired softness.

b. While eggs are cooking, heat rice and blended vegetables in a separate bowl in the microwave for 2 minutes.

c. Join all ingredients in a medium bowl, adding soy sauce or other Asian sauce exactly as you would prefer.

Per Serving

- Calories: 187
- Fat: 1g Protein: 11g
- Sodium: 202mg
- Fiber: 3g
- Carbohydrates: 35g
- Sugar: 0g

28. Lemon-Herb Grilled Chicken Salad

This is a fresh take on a flame-broiled salad—exceptionally refreshing, and ideal for the late spring when you would prefer not to turn your oven on. Garnish this with a cut of fresh lemon if desired.

Ingredients

Serves 1

- 4 ounces flame-broiled chicken breast, cut
- 1 cup blended greens
- 1 tablespoon olive oil
- 1 tablespoon lemon juice
- ½ teaspoon garlic salt

- ¼ teaspoon rosemary

Advantages of Lemon Juice

Lemons are very alkalizing for your body, which means they help maintain a stable pH balance. In the body, you have a certain degree of acidity, called the pH balance. A lot of acidities can cause fatigue, muscular cramping and pain, and brevity of breath. Lemons are also good for the liver, an important organ in the body that acts as a detoxifying organ. Lemon is a natural cleansing agent, and it can help bolster the liver in its push to detoxify your bloodstream.

Direction

In a medium bowl, put all the ingredients together.

Per Serving

- Calories: 314
- Fat: 17g
- Protein: 30g
- Sodium: 146mg
- Fiber: 7g
- Carbohydrates: 12g
- Sugar: 4g

29. Pulled Chicken BBQ Sandwich

This dish is a tasty and easy way to give a punch to destroyed chicken. You can utilize any sauce you like, including barbecue, hot wing, ranch, or whatever your favorite sauce maybe.

Ingredients

Serves 1

- 4 ounces destroyed chicken, warmed
- 2 tablespoons barbecue sauce, or any sauce of decision
- 1 whole-wheat hamburger bun

Direction

a. In a medium bowl, blend warm destroyed chicken and barbecue sauce, making sure to coat chicken in the sauce.

b. Place heated chicken and sauce blend on a hamburger bun and serve.

Per Serving

- Calories: 349
- Fat: 18g
- Protein: 21g
- Sodium: 605mg
- Fiber: 1g
- Carbohydrates: 24g
- Sugar: 9g

30. Sausage and Spicy Eggs

This is a beautiful dish that isn't just a delectable breakfast but is also suitable for lunch or a late dinner. Be careful not to utilize an excessive salt; most sausages have a considerable amount of salt, so taste first.

Ingredients

Serves 4

- 1-pound Italian sweet sausage

- ¼ cup water 1 tablespoon olive oil
- 2 mediums red chile peppers, roasted and chopped
- 1 medium jalapeño, seeded and minced
- 8 large whole eggs
- ¾ cup 2% milk 2 tablespoons fresh parsley for garnish Protein Variations

Feel allowed to utilize 1 pound of turkey sausage, regular breakfast sausage, ground hamburger, or even disintegrated bacon instead of the Italian sausage for this recipe.

Direction

a. Cut the sausage into ¼" coins. Place them in a heavy skillet with the water and olive oil. Heat to the point of boiling; at that point, turn down the heat to stew.

b. When the sausages are earthy colored, expel them and place them on a paper towel. Add the sweet red peppers and the jalapeño to the pan, and sauté them over medium heat for 5 minutes.

c. While the peppers are sautéing, beat the eggs and milk together enthusiastically.

d. Add the blend to the pan and tenderly crease it over until it is puffed and soggy.

e. Mix in the saved sausage, garnish with parsley and serve hot.

Per Serving

- Calories: 383
- Fat: 23g
- Protein: 35g
- Sodium: 89mg
- Fiber: 2g

- Carbohydrates: 8g
- Sugar: 2g

31. Lentil Salad

This is a salad with an explosion of protein. Serve it as a main lunch course or as aside.

Ingredients

Serves 4

- (1-pound) bag lentils (green, yellow, or red)
- 1 medium onion, stripped and chopped
- ½ cup wine vinegar
- ½ teaspoon salt
- 1 medium carrot, stripped and diced
- 2 medium stalks celery, chopped
- 2 medium tomatoes,
- cut 1 cup French Dressing (see sidebar)

French Dressing

- In a blender, blend ⅓ cup red wine vinegar;
- ½ teaspoon Worcestershire sauce;
- 1 clove garlic, chopped;
- tablespoons chopped fresh parsley;
- 1 teaspoon dried thyme; and
- 1 teaspoon dried rosemary.

Slowly add ⅔ cup extra-virgin olive oil in a meager stream with the goal that the ingredients will emulsify.

Direction

a. Cover the lentils with water in a small saucepan and add the onions and wine vinegar. Heat to the boiling point, lower the heat, and stew until the lentils are soft, about 45 minutes. Sprinkle with salt.

b. Toss with the diced carrot and chopped celery and then arrange the tomatoes around the hill of lentils. Sprinkle with French Dressing and serve warm or at room temperature.

Per Serving
- Calories: 287
- Fat: 20g
- Protein: 7g
- Sodium: 631mg
- Fiber: 27g
- Carbohydrates: 25g
- Sugar: 6g

32. Portobello Mushroom Salad with Gorgonzola, Peppers, and Bacon

The hot Gorgonzola cheese separates this salad as an impressive lunch.

Ingredients Serve 4
- 2 large portobello mushrooms.
- ½ cup French Dressing
- 4 strips bacon
- 4 ounces Gorgonzola cheese, disintegrated
- ½cup mayonnaise 2 cups chopped romaine lettuce

- ½ cup chopped roasted red pepper

Mushroom Choice

There are many varieties of mushrooms available. Earthy colored mushrooms have a vigorous flavor. White button mushrooms are flavorful in sauces, and the large ones work well when stuffed or flame-broiled. Get wild mushrooms from a reputable mycologist. Never surmise if a wild mushroom that you find in the forested areas is safe. It may be harmful!

Direction

a. Marinate the mushrooms for 1 hour in the French Dressing. Fry the bacon in a small skillet over medium heat until fresh; set it on paper towels and disintegrate it.

b. On a hot flame broil or in an oven, barbecue the mushrooms for 3 minutes.

c. Cut them into strips.

d. While the mushrooms are cooking, heat the Gorgonzola and mayonnaise in a small saucepan on low until the cheese liquefies.

e. Place the mushrooms on the bed of lettuce. Sprinkle with the bacon.

f. Sprinkle with the cheese blend and garnish with roasted red peppers.

Per Serving

- Calories: 365
- Fat: 31g
- Protein: 11g
- Sodium: 413mg
- Fiber: 12g
- Carbohydrates: 12g
- Sugar: 3g

33. Asparagus Salad with Hard-Boiled Egg

This is an exquisite salad to serve during the all-too-brief asparagus season. For an easy variation, hurl in some extra cooked or smoked salmon.

Ingredients

- Serves 4
- 3 tablespoons olive oil 1½ pounds steamed asparagus
- 2 large hard-boiled eggs, coarsely grated
- 2 tablespoons lemon juice
- 3 tablespoons white wine vinegar
- ½ teaspoon Dijon mustard
- ½ tablespoon lemon pizzazz 2 tablespoons minced fresh dill
- 1 tablespoon minced Italian parsley
- ¼ teaspoon sea salt

Direction

The Perfect Hard-Boiled Egg
- a. Place eggs in a pan with a top. Fill the pan with cold water until it is ¾"– 1" above the eggs.
- b. Allow boiling. Expel from heat and spread, let the eggs sit for 15 minutes. Drain and run under cool water, use immediately or refrigerate.

c. In a large bowl, hurl together the asparagus and eggs. Put in a safe spot.

d. In another bowl, flutter the vinegar, oil, mustard, lemon juice, lemon get-up-and-go, dill, parsley, and salt. Sprinkle over the asparagus and egg. Hurl delicately. Serve immediately.

Per Serving
- Calories: 167
- Fat: 13g
- Protein: 7g
- Sodium: 194mg
- Fiber: 4g
- Carbohydrates: 8g
- Sugar: 3g

CHAPTER NINE; DINNER: BEEF, PORK, AND POULTRY

34. Baked Buffalo Chicken Strips

Here is a healthy and flavorful alternative to the ever-popular buffalo wings. Make certain to check your wing sauce; many are low in calories, but some are made with butter, sugar, or other calorie-thick ingredients. The Homemade Buffalo Wing Sauce is a great alternative.

Ingredients

Serves 4

- 1 teaspoon ground black pepper
- ½ cup flour or flour substitute
- 1-pound chicken strips
- 1 teaspoon ground cayenne pepper
- ½ cup buffalo wing sauce

Direction

a. Preheat oven to around 450°F, and line a 13" × 9" baking pan with aluminum foil.
b. In a large bowl or zip-top bag, join black pepper, cayenne, and flour. Add chicken fingers and hurl together until chicken is secured.

c. Lay chicken fingers on prepared pan and cook 30–40 minutes or until juices run clear, flipping halfway through.
   d. Remove from oven, pour buffalo sauce over tenders, and serve.

Per Serving

- Calories: 196
- Fat: 4g Protein: 26g
- Sodium: 832mg
- Fiber: 1g
- Carbohydrates: 13g
- Sugar: 0g

35. Un-Dried Tomato Stuffed Chicken

This tasty recipe is overflowing with flavor. Make certain to get regular chicken breasts, not dainty cut, so that they can be cut as required.

Ingredients

Serves 4

- 1-pound boneless, skinless chicken breast
- ½ cup feta cheese 1
- (3.5-ounce) package sun-dried tomatoes
- 2 tablespoons pesto
- ¼ teaspoon salt
- ¼ teaspoon pepper

Direction

Preheat oven to 350°F.

a. Butterfly chicken breast by cutting the long way. You want the chicken to overlay open like a book; you don't want it chopped into two separate pieces.

b. Lay feta cheese, tomatoes, and pesto down one half of chicken breast. Overlap chicken back over itself, utilizing a toothpick to seal if necessary, and place in glass baking dish.

c. Season the chicken with pepper and salt, and bake 35–40 minutes, or until juices run clear.

Per Serving
- Calories: 271 Fat: 9g
- Protein: 29g
- Sodium: 951mg
- Fiber: 3g
- Carbohydrates: 12g
- Sugar: 12g

36. Chicken and Bean Burrito

This recipe calls for cooking in a microwave, which is great for those days when you are in a surge. If you'd like, you can add harsh low-fat cream to the completed burrito.

Ingredients
Serves 1
- ½ cup cooked pinto beans
- 2 teaspoons taco seasoning
- 2 tablespoons medium salsa
- 3 ounces cooked chicken 1 (8") whole-wheat tortilla

- 2 tablespoons low-fat cheese

Direction

a. Add pinto beans, taco seasoning, and salsa to a food processor and mix.

b. Place blend along with the cooked chicken into a tortilla, and sprinkle the cheese on top.

c. Microwave 15–25 seconds, or heat in the oven until cheese is liquefied.

Per Serving

- Calories: 404
- Fat: 11g
- Protein: 33g
- Sodium: 1,750mg
- Fiber: 9g Carbohydrates: 44g
- Sugar: 5g

37. Tamarind Pot Roast

Fresh tamarind units have a fresh, splendid taste that livens up any pot roast.

Ingredients

Serves 8

- 2½ pounds top round roast
- 1 teaspoon salt
- 1 teaspoon paprika 1 cup flour 2 tablespoons canola oil
- 2 medium onions, chopped
- 1 teaspoon freshly ground black pepper

- 4 cloves garlic, minced 1" handle ginger, minced
- 2 large carrots, cut into coins
- 2 cups of meat stock
- 4 tamarind units, skin cut
- ¼ cup lemon juice
- 2 tablespoons dark soy sauce

38. Terrific Tamarind

Tamarind comes in earthy colored, papery-looking cases with soft, consumable earthy glowing mash; it has a harsh, sweet taste; it is utilized in a variety of candies, sauces, squeezes, and jams. In Ayurvedic medication, tamarind is used to treat digestive issues.

Direction
   a. 1.Preheat oven to 350°F.
   b. Season the pot roast with salt, pepper, and paprika.
   c. Sprinkle the flour on a plate. Dig the roast in the flour.
   d. Heat the oil in a Dutch oven. Earthy colored the hamburger on all sides. Evacuate to a secured dish. Add the onion, garlic, ginger, and carrots to the Dutch oven. Sauté 5 minutes.
   e. Meanwhile, heat the stock and tamarind to the point of boiling in a small saucepan, blending much of the time.
   f. Return the meat to the Dutch oven. Whisk the tamarind blend through a strainer over the hamburger. Add the lemon juice and soy sauce. Heat to the point of boiling.
   g. Place Dutch oven into the oven—cover and bake for 2½ hours.

Per Serving

- Calories: 310
- Fat: 9g Protein: 36g
- Sodium: 738mg
- Fiber: 2g
- Carbohydrates: 19g
- Sugar: 3g

39. Mustard Pecan Chicken

You can utilize any nuts in this recipe, but pecans work especially well.

Ingredients

Serves 4

- ½ cup shelled pecans
- 2 tablespoons Dijon mustard
- 2 tablespoons nonfat plain Greek yogurt (4-ounce) boneless, skinless chicken breasts
- 1 tablespoon macadamia oil

Direction

a. Place pecans in a food processor and crush until they're a medium-fine consistency.
b. In a small bowl, combine mustard and yogurt, mixing well.
c. Lay chicken breasts on a plate and spread half the mustard and yogurt blend on one side. Sprinkle half the ground pecans over mustard blend and press daintily with the back of a spoon to enable them to stick.

d. Coat a large skillet with macadamia oil and place over medium-high heat. Add chicken, pecan-side down, and cook about 4 minutes. With chicken still in the pan, spread the remaining mustard-yogurt blend on the sides.

e. Sprinkle remaining pecans on top by pressing them in a piece with the back of a spoon.

f. Flip breasts over carefully, doing your best not to unstick the covering.

g. Cook another 5 minutes and serve.

Per Serving

- Calories: 262
- Fat: 17g
- Protein: 26g
- Sodium: 222mg
- Fiber: 2g Carbohydrates: 3g
- Sugar: 1g

40. Papaya Pulled Pork

Papaya gives dampness, body, and flavor to this tropical pulled pork.

Ingredients

Serves 8

- 1 (3-pound) boneless pork shoulder roast, cut back of excess
- 3 cups cubed papaya, stripped
- 2 tablespoons ginger juice
- ¼ cup pineapple juice
- ¼ cup tomato paste

- 3 serrano peppers,
- diced 1 medium onion,
- diced 5 cloves garlic,
- cut 1 tablespoon yellow hot sauce
- 1 teaspoon of sea salt
- 1 teaspoon bean stew powder
- 1 teaspoon paprika

Direction

a. Arrange all ingredients in a 4-quart then reduce the cooker. Cook on low for 8–10 hours.
b. Remove the meat and pull apart with forks. Mash any solids in the slow cooker with a potato masher.
c. Set the meat back to the pan, then slow the cooker and mix to join.

Per Serving Calories: 297

- Fat: 12g
- Protein: 34g
- Sodium: 243mg
- Fiber: 2g
- Carbohydrates: 11g
- Sugar: 5g

41. Pesto Pork Chops

You can utilize the guidelines in this recipe to make the pesto, or if you already have Basil Pesto you can save time and use that.

Ingredients

Serves 4

- 2 cloves garlic
- ¼ cup fresh basil leaves
- ¼ cup fresh parsley leaves
- Zest of ½ large lemon
- 2 tablespoons water
- 1 tablespoon olive oil
- ¼ teaspoon salt
- (4-ounce) pork cleaves, cut back of excess

Direction

a. First, make the pesto: Place garlic in a food processor and heartbeat until chopped. Add basil, parsley, and lemon pizzazz and heartbeat until chopped.

b. Add water, olive oil, and salt, at that point procedure until almost smooth—transfer to serving dish.

c. Add pork slashes to a large skillet over medium-high heat and cook for about 5minutes for each side or until cooked through.

d. Coat the pork hacks with nearly half of the pesto blend as they prepare, coating each side before turning.

e. Remove pork cleaves to a serving dish and present it with the remaining pesto.

Per Serving

- Calories: 182
- Fat: 8g
- Protein: 25g
- Sodium: 215mg
- Fiber: 0g
- Carbohydrates: 1g
- Sugar: 0g

42. Argentinian Steak

A delightful turn on a traditional sirloin that makes certain to please; this dish works out positively for a side salad or garlicky greens.

Ingredients

Serves 2

- 2 tablespoons water
- ½ cup chopped fresh parsley leaves
- ½ cup chopped fresh cilantro leaves
- 1 tablespoon lemon juice
- 1 tablespoon olive oil
- ¼ teaspoon salt
- ¼ teaspoon ground black pepper
- ½ teaspoon red pepper flakes
- 2 (4-ounce) sirloin steaks

Which Steak to Use?

Steaks will vary cut by cut, so there is no clear best steak alternative. If you want lower fat, generally, sirloin will be a good alternative. If you prefer a little progressively fat and flavor, the rib eye is the right decision.

Direction

a. Combine water, parsley, cilantro, lemon juice, oil, salt, black pepper, and red pepper in a large bowl.
b. Place steak on flame broil rack or skillet over medium-high heat and cook about 4 minutes for each side.
c. Place the steak to the chopping board and allow it to stand 10 minutes.
d. Thinly cut steaks across the grain. Blend in with parsley and cilantro blend.
e. Serve and Enjoy.

Per Serving

- Calories: 222
- Fat: 13g
- Protein: 24g
- Sodium: 372mg
- Fiber: 1g
- Carbohydrates: 2g
- Sugar: 0g

43. Lean Meat Balls

This recipe utilizes lean meat, but you can also use ground turkey or chicken. These go well served over whole-grain spaghetti and marinara sauce or are delightful without anyone else with a side of steamed green vegetables.

Ingredients

Serves 6

- 1-pound extra-lean ground meat
- ½ cup minced onion
- 2 large egg whites
- 1 large whole egg
- ¼ cup oat bran
- 2 tablespoons low-fat grated Parmesan cheese
- 1 teaspoon dried oregano
- ½ teaspoon garlic powder
- 2 tablespoons skim milk
- ¼ teaspoon salt
- ¼ teaspoon ground black pepper

Direction

a. Heat oven to 375°F.
b. In a large bowl, combine all ingredients.
c. Shape into balls generally the size of golfballs; you ought to have 20 meatballs total.
d. Bake 25 minutes on a 13" × 9" baking sheet.

Per Serving

- Calories: 174
- Fat: 9g
- Protein: 18g
- Sodium: 187mg
- Fiber: 1g
- Carbohydrates: 5g

- Sugar: 1g

44. Tuscan Chicken

Here is a flavorful, slow-cooked chicken recipe that stores well and presents a variety of side dishes.

Ingredients
- Serves 4 ¼ cups chopped onion
- ½ medium red ringer pepper, seeded and cut into strips
- ½ medium green ringer pepper, seeded and cut into strips
- 1 (8-ounce) can black beans, drained
- (4-ounce) boneless, skinless chicken breasts
- 2 tablespoons olive oil
- 1 large tomato, diced
- ¼ cup low-sodium chicken stock
- 1 tablespoon apple juice vinegar
- ½ teaspoon dried oregano
- 1 clove garlic, squashed
- ¼ teaspoon salt

Direction
a. Place onion, peppers, and beans in a slow cooker.
b. Place chicken on vegetables and beans.
c. In a medium bowl, mix olive oil, tomato, stock, vinegar, oregano, garlic, and salt. Pour blend over the chicken in the slow cooker.
d. Set the cooker on low heat. Cook 6–7 hours, until chicken is not, at this point, pink, at that point, serve.

Per Serving

- Calories: 263
- Fat: 10g
- Protein: 28g
- Sodium: 513mg
- Fiber: 4g
- Carbohydrates: 14g
- Sugar: 4g

45. Lager Can Chicken

The lager in this chicken just adds dampness—you won't taste it at all. If you choose to evade alcohol, you can utilize a can of Coca-Cola. The calories for both are generally the same, and the chicken won't absorb quite a bit of it anyway, so you don't have to stress a lot over tallying calories.

Ingredients

Serves 6

- 1 (4-pound) whole chicken
- 2 tablespoons olive oil
- 1 tablespoon ground black pepper
- 2 tablespoons sliced fresh thyme leaves or 1 tablespoon dried thyme
- 1 tablespoon fit salt
- 1 half-full 12-ounce can brew, opened and at room temperature

Direction

a. Remove some parts like the neck and giblets from the cavity of the chicken. Rub chicken all finished with olive oil.

b. In a small bowl, consolidate salt, pepper, and thyme. Sprinkle blend over chicken.

c. Make sure brew can is just half-loaded up with lager, with cuts cut into the top of the can with a knife. Lower chicken into the open container, so the chicken is sitting upstanding with the container in its cavity.

d. Place chicken on a flame broil, utilizing the legs, and lager can act as a tripod to sustenance the chicken and keep it firm.

e. Cover flame broil. Try not to check the chicken for at least 60 minutes. After 60 minutes, start checking chicken at regular intervals or somewhere in the vicinity, until a meat thermometer embedded into the deepest part of the thigh shows 160°F–165°F.

f. Delicately transfer chicken to a tray or pan; let rest 10 minutes, at that point serve.

Per Serving

- Calories: 410
- Fat: 13g
- Protein: 64g
- Sodium: 1,411mg
- Fiber: 0g
- Carbohydrates: 2g
- Sugar: 0g

46. Steakhouse Blue Cheese Burger

This tasty burger can be enjoyed without anyone else with a side of greens or served on a hamburger bun.

Ingredients

Serves 4

- 1 pound lean ground meat
- 1 large whole egg
- ¼ cup bread pieces
- 1 tablespoon McCormick Grill Mates Classic Steakhouse Burger Seasoning
- ½ cup blue cheese disintegrates

Direction

a. In a large bowl, consolidate meat, egg, bread pieces, and seasoning. Blend well.
b. Form into 4 equally shaped patties.
c. Place patties on flame broil (or in the skillet) and cook to desired doneness, approximately 4–5 minutes for each side.
d. After the first flip, sprinkle blue cheese disintegrates on the patties and allow them to dissolve as it cooks.

Per Serving

- Calories: 257
- Fat: 12g
- Protein: 30g
- Sodium: 367mg
- Fiber: 0g
- Carbohydrates: 5g

- Sugar: 1g

47. Spaghetti Marinara with Chicken and Basil

This ameliorating dish is ideal for a high-carb day. If you're searching for a lower-carb alternative, substitute cooked spaghetti squash or zucchini noodles for the pasta.

Ingredients It serves 6

- 3 tablespoons of olive oil, separated
- 2 small yellow onions,
- stripped and diced 2 cloves garlic,
- minced ½ cup red wine
- 1 (28-ounce) can squashed tomatoes
- 3 teaspoons salt, divided
- 2 teaspoons freshly ground black pepper, isolated
- 2 teaspoons dried oregano or Italian seasoning
- ¾ pound (12 ounces) spaghetti 1 pound chicken tenders
- ½ cup basil leaves, torn or left whole
- ½ cup freshly destroyed Parmesan cheese

Versatile Marinara

This speedy marinara sauce is easily adapted to suit your taste or your desired dish. Swap the red wine for hamburger stock for a more profound, heartier flavor and present with meatballs. Add in diced carrot, celery, or red and green chime pepper while sautéing the onions for added flavor, nourishment, and crunch. Adding cinnamon and allspice gives the sauce a Greek flair; serve beat with disintegrated feta instead of Parmesan. Sautéed or flame-broiled shrimp and scallops make an elegant pairing with this basic sauce. Experiment and discover what you enjoy!

Direction

a. To prepare the marinara, heat 2 tablespoons olive oil in a medium skillet or, on the other hand, small Dutch oven over medium heat. At the point when oil is sparkling, add onions.

b. Sauté onions, occasionally mixing, until they are soft and translucent, about 15 minutes. Be certain onions aren't charring; if they start to consume, turn the heat down.

c. Once onions are translucent and soft, add garlic and cook until fragrant, 1–2 minutes progressively, blending to make sure nothing consumes.

d. Pour wine into pan and heat to high. Boil until wine lessens by half, scraping the earthy colored bits from the base of the pan to release flavor.

e. Add tomatoes and mix to join. Add 1 teaspoon pepper, 2 teaspoons salt, and oregano and mix. Lessen heat to low, and stew 20 minutes.

f. While sauce is stewing, heat a large pot of water to the point of boiling. Add spaghetti and allow to cook until al dente, according to package directions. Drain, place back into the hot pot, and coat with 1 tablespoon oil, so the pasta doesn't stick.

g. Preheat a nonstick barbecue pan over medium-high heat. Season chicken on the two sides with 1 teaspoon salt and 1 teaspoon pepper.

h. When the pan is heated, sear chicken 5 minutes, until chicken turns white and barbecue marks appear. Flip and flame broil 4–5 minutes more, or just until the internal temperature reaches 165°F.

i. To serve, isolate warm spaghetti among six plates or serving bowls. Top with marinara, and settle chicken pieces on top or as an afterthought. Scatter basil leaves and sprinkle with cheese.

Per Serving

- Calories: 483
- Fat: 15g
- Protein: 31g
- Sodium: 1,728mg
- Fiber: 4g
- Carbohydrates: 51g
- Sugar: 6g

48. Lean Turkey Meatloaf

This straightforward recipe is a fantastic low-fat, high-protein choice. Pair it with vegetables on your low-carb days, and serve it with a side of rice or mashed potatoes on a high-carb day.

Ingredients

Serves 4

- 1½ pounds lean ground turkey
- ¼ cup bread scraps

- 1 sizeable whole egg
- ½ medium onion, stripped and grated
- 2 tablespoons milk
- ½ teaspoon salt
- ½ teaspoon ground black pepper
- 2 tablespoons ketchup

Direction

a. Preheat oven to 450°F.

b. In a large bowl, consolidate turkey, bread pieces, egg, onion, milk, salt, and pepper. Try not to overwork. Structure into a loaf and place on a baking sheet or in a 9" × 5" bread pan.

c. Brush top with ketchup; at that point, cook 30–35 minutes before serving. Meat should reach an inner temperature of about 165°F.

Per Serving
- Calories: 313
- Fat: 16g
- Protein: 32g
- Sodium: 607mg
- Fiber: 1g
- Carbohydrates: 9g
- Sugar: 3g

49. Marinated Grilled Turkey Cutlets

If you're serving this on a high-carb day, flame broils some fresh corn alongside the turkey for an easy side dish; they cook in about the same amount of time.

Ingredients

Serves 6

- 6 thick-cut turkey breast cutlets
- 1 cup light coconut milk
- 1 medium onion,
- diced 4 cloves garlic,
- minced 1 small Scotch cap pepper,
- minced, seeds expelled
- 2 tablespoons canola oil
- 1 tablespoon Caribbean-style curry powder
- 1 teaspoon fresh thyme leaves
- 1/2 teaspoon ground cayenne
- 1/2 teaspoon hot paprika
- 1/4 teaspoon freshly grated nutmeg
- 1 teaspoon of sea salt

Why Use Fresh Herbs?

Fresh herbs have a greater amount of the original nutrients intact than dried. The flavor of fresh

herbs is more brilliant than dried herbs. Fresh herbs also add the measurement of flavor to recipes.

Direction

a. Set all ingredients in a marinating vessel or resealable plastic bag. Seal and shake to distribute the ingredients. Refrigerate a minimum of 1 hour or as long as 8 hours.

b. Prepare your flame broil according to the manufacturer's directions. Grease the flame broil grate. Expel the turkey from the marinade. Discard the marinade.

c. Grill, flipping once until wholly cooked (165°F), about 10 minutes.

Per Serving
- Calories: 255
- Fat: 14g
- Protein: 29g
- Sodium: 455mg
- Fiber: 1g
- Carbohydrates: 5g
- Sugar: 1g

50. Garlic-Studded Pork Roast

Embeddings garlic into the roast, not just mixes it with flavor; it keeps the meat sodden as well.

Ingredients

Serves 8

- 1 (2-pound) pork midsection
- 1 head garlic, stripped
- 1 cup basil
- 1 cup Italian parsley
- 2 tablespoons olive oil
- ¼ cup lemon juice
- 2 tablespoons lemon get-up-and-go
- 1 teaspoon sea salt
- 1 teaspoon freshly ground black pepper

Garlic's Many Uses

Garlic is a fundamental fixing in thousands of dishes around the world. Traditionally, garlic has been utilized to treat the basic virus. It also has antibacterial activity and has been used as an antiseptic.

Direction

a. Preheat oven to 350°F.
b. Cut cuts on all sides of the midsection and supplement a garlic clove in each one.
c. Place the basil, parsley, olive oil, lemon juice, lemon pizzazz, salt, and enthusiasm per in a food processor. Heartbeat until a paste structure.

d. Rub the paste over the pork. Place in a Dutch oven and roast for 40 minutes or until the pork is completely cooked, reaching an internal temperature between 145°F (medium-rare) and 160°F (medium). Allow pork to rest 5–10 minutes before cutting and serving.

Per Serving
- Calories: 191
- Fat: 10g
- Protein: 24g
- Sodium: 357mg
- Fiber: 0g
- Carbohydrates: 2g
- Sugar: 0g

CHAPER TEN; DINNER: FISH AND SHELLFISH

51. Dijon Tuna

A basic and flavorful way to prepare tuna steaks; you may have the option to discover fresh tuna steaks at a local market if you live near the water. Something else, check your local health foods store to discover quality steaks.

Ingredients

Serves

- 2 tablespoons Dijon mustard
- 1 teaspoon Worcestershire sauce
- 1 teaspoon lemon juice
- ¼ teaspoon sea salt
- 2 (6-ounce) tuna steaks

Pick Your Fish

This recipe works out positively for tuna, but you can also substitute cod, salmon, tilapia, or any other fish you have. It will, at present, taste tasty.

Direction

a. Preheat oven to 375°F.

b. In a medium bowl, consolidate the mustard, Worcestershire sauce, lemon squeeze, and salt. Blend well.

c. Place tuna steaks on a 13" × 9" baking sheet and pour mustard blend over them, making sure to coat the fish.

d. Bake up to 15 to 20 minutes or until fish flakes easily with a fork.

Per Serving

- Calories: 255
- Fat: 9g
- Protein: 40g
- Sodium: 566mg
- Fiber: 1g
- Carbohydrates: 2g
- Sugar: 0g

52. Coconut Garlic Shrimp

This can be filled in as a side dish with another meal or enjoyed as a meal, ultimately all alone, perhaps with a side salad or bowl of greens.

Ingredients

Serves 2

- 1 tablespoon coconut oil
- 2 cloves garlic, minced
- 2 shallots, minced
- 8 ounces thawed shrimp, shelled and deveined
- 2 tablespoons destroyed coconut, raw if conceivable
- 1 tablespoon lemon juice

- 1 tablespoon chopped dill

Direction

a. Heat coconut oil in an average skillet over medium heat.
b. Add garlic and shallots and sauté about 2 minutes.
c. Add shrimp and cook 3 minutes.
d. Add remaining ingredients, mix about 1 minute, and serve.

Per Serving

- Calories: 216
- Fat: 10g
- Protein: 23g
- Sodium: 330mg
- Fiber: 1g
- Carbohydrates: 7g
- Sugar: 1g

53. Shrimp-Orange Kebabs

The citrus–soy sauce makes these shrimp kebabs sing.

Ingredients

Serves 4

- 1 large navel orange,
- halved and cut into wedges
- 1 large red onion, cut into wedges
- 1-pound large shrimp, stripped and deveined
- 2 tablespoons orange juice
- 2 tablespoons soy sauce

Speared

Pick sticks that have one pointy end. Stick the food straightforwardly in the middle. Each bit of food on the stick ought to be of similar size for flame broiling.

Direction

a. Heat barbecue to medium. Oil the flame broil rack.
b. Thread the orange wedges, onion, and shrimp on 4 sticks, starting and finishing with oranges.
c. In a small bowl, whisk both the orange juice and soy sauce. Brush the sauce over the sticks.
d. Grill kebabs until the shrimp are completely cooked, about 5 minutes total.

Per Serving

- Calories: 153
- Fat: 2g
- Protein: 24g
- Sodium: 616mg
- Fiber: 1g
- Carbohydrates: 9g
- Sugar: 5g

54. Spinach and Feta Salmon

A tasty supper is packed with healthy fats; you can use lower-fat choices for the yogurt and cheese if you want to lower the total calories in the meal.

Ingredients

Serves 2

- 2 tablespoons plain Greek yogurt
- ¼ cup disintegrated feta cheese 1 scallion, cut across
- ¼ cup chopped fresh spinach
- 1 teaspoon olive oil 2 (6-ounce) salmon fillets

Direction

a. Preheat oven to 350°F.
b. In a medium bowl, join yogurt, cheese, scallion, spinach, and olive oil. Blend well in with a fork.
c. Spread the blend uniformly over filets.
d. Place fillets in an 8" × 8" glass baking dish and bake 15 minutes.

Per Serving

- Calories: 319
- Fat: 17g
- Protein: 37g
- Sodium: 294mg
- Fiber: 0g
- Carbohydrates: 2g
- Sugar: 2g

55. Stuffed Salmon Filets

A tasty way to serve salmon, with marginally less fat than the Spinach and Feta Salmon recipe is in this chapter.

Ingredients

Serves 2

- 2 (6-ounce) salmon fillets
- 1 large lemon, meagerly cut
- 1 scallion, cut
- 1 tablespoon dried oregano
- 1 tablespoon dried thyme

Wild-Caught Salmon versus Farm Raised

While it is increasingly expensive, wild-caught salmon is the better alternative if you can afford it. Wild salmon will swim in its natural environment, eating a well-adjusted diet, while farm-raised salmon are regularly taken care of a restricted food sup-handle. To get a healthier fat profile, go with wild-caught when you can.

Direction

a. Preheat oven to 425°F.
b. Slice salmon horizontally about ⅔ of the way through.
c. Stuff filets with lemon slices, scallions, oregano, and thyme.
d. Place the stuffed fillets in a 9" × 9" glass baking dish and bake 15 minutes.

Per Serving

- Calories: 255
- Fat: 10g Protein: 34g
- Sodium: 77mg
- Fiber: 2g
- Carbohydrates: 5g
- Sugar: 1g

56. Salmon Burgers

Canned fish is readily available at most stores, while fresh fish can sometimes be hard to get. This recipe for salmon patties is easy to prepare and offers variety from the standard baked fish or regular burgers.

Ingredients

Serves 2

- 1 (8-ounce) can salmon, drained
- 1 large whole egg Dash onion powder
- 2 tablespoons dry oats or bread scraps
- 1 teaspoon olive oil

Dietary Fats

Concerning dietary fats, we traditionally hear about good fats and bad fats. This alludes to the nutritional breakdown, as the two sorts of fat will at present have 9 calories for each gram. Good fats are usually higher in omega-3s, are anti-inflammatory, and incorporate avocado, whole eggs, and fat cuts of fish. Bad fats, in general, are higher in omega-6s, can cause inflammation, and incorporate prepared and seared foods and trans fats.

Direction

a. Mix all ingredients aside from the olive oil in a large bowl, mashing together with a fork. Structure blend into 2 patties.
b. Heat oil in a average skillet over medium heat; add the patties.
c. Cook about 4 minutes for every side, carefully turning with a spatula.

Per Serving

- Calories: 265
- Fat: 13g Protein: 30g
- Sodium: 439mg
- Fiber: 1g
- Carbohydrates: 5g
- Sugar: 0g

57. Sun-Dried Tomato Tuna

This dish can be eaten alone or presented with chips or celery for plunging. A great meal without anyone else, or you can share it as an appetizer.

Ingredients Serve 1

- 1 tablespoon olive oil
- 2 tablespoons sun-dried tomatoes
- ½ teaspoon dried parsley
- 1 clove garlic, minced
- ¼ teaspoon salt
- ⅛ teaspoon ground black pepper
- 4 ounces canned tuna, flushed and drained

Direction

a. Add olive oil, sun-dried tomatoes, parsley, garlic, salt, and pepper to a blender and mix until it shapes a paste.

b. Place tuna in a bowl and pour the sun-dried tomato blend over the top. Blend to consolidate. Fill in as is, or warm in the oven or microwave first.

Per Serving
- Calories: 328
- Fat: 22g
- Protein: 27g
- Sodium: 1,135mg
- Fiber: 1g Carbohydrates: 5g
- Sugar: 3g

58. Lemon and Garlic Cod Filets

Here is a straightforward, speedy, and lean way to get some fish in your diet. This works out positively for a garlicky blended greens dish as an afterthought.

Ingredients

Serves 2

- 1 clove garlic, minced
- 1 tablespoon olive oil 2 (6-ounce) cod fillets
- 1 tablespoon lemon pepper
- ¼ teaspoon garlic salt Juice from ½ large fresh lemon

Direction
a. Preheat oven to 400°F.
b. In a small bowl, blend garlic and olive oil and brush blend over both sides of fish and place the fish in an oiled glass 9" × 9" baking dish.
c. Sprinkle fish with lemon pepper and garlic salt. Sprinkle with lemon juice.

d. Bake up to 10 to 15 minutes, or until fish flakes easily.

Per Serving

- Calories: 257
- Fat: 8g
- Protein: 41g
- Sodium: 420mg
- Fiber: 0g
- Carbohydrates: 2g
- Sugar: 0g

59. Shrimp Scampi

This classic dish gives a tasty way to get some carbs if presented with pasta, and the shrimp is a great wellspring of lean protein. It very well may be presented with greens for a low-carb alternative or over a bed of pasta for a higher-carb meal.

Ingredients

Serves 2

- 1 tablespoon butter
- 4 cloves garlic, minced
- 1 shallot, chopped
- 1 pound raw large shrimp, stripped and deveined
- ¼ teaspoon salt
- ⅛ teaspoon ground black pepper
- 2 tablespoons lemon juice
- 3 tablespoons white wine

Direction

a. In a big pan, heat butter over average-high heat and sauté garlic and shallots 2 minutes.

b. Add shrimp and sprinkle with pepper and salt. Let it cook for 3–4 minutes.

c. Add the lemon squeeze and white wine; combine it all: Cook 1–2 minutes before serving.

Per Serving

- Calories: 339
- Fat: 10g
- Protein: 46g
- Sodium: 635mg
- Fiber: 0g
- Carbohydrates: 10g
- Sugar: 1g

60. Firm Parmesan Fish Sticks

These delectable fish sticks give a high-protein, low-fat meal. Present with your plunging sauce of decision or eat plain.

Ingredients

Serves

- 4 ½ cup panko bread pieces
- 2 tablespoons flour or flour substitute
- ¼ cup grated Parmesan cheese
- 1 tablespoon Italian seasoning
- 2 large egg whites
- 1 pound tilapia, cut into long strips

The Leanest Fish?

In general, white fish, such as cod, halibut, and tilapia, will be lower in fat and have fewer calories. This is good when watching calories. For example, higher-fat fish, tuna or salmon, have more calories but also increasingly good omega-3 fatty acids. The decision is yours.

Direction
- a. Preheat oven to 400°F.
- b. In a shallow bowl, consolidate bread morsels, flour, cheese, and seasoning. Place egg whites in a separate shallow bowl.
- c. Dip fish strips into egg whites; then, move in the dry blend to coat and place on a baking sheet.
- d. Once all strips have been coated, bake 15 minutes and serve.

Per Serving
- Calories: 258
- Fat: 4g
- Protein: 28g
- Sodium: 670mg
- Fiber: 2g
- Carbohydrates: 25g
- Sugar: 3g

61. Feta and Tuna Pasta Salad

This protein and carb blend is rich **whe**n eaten fresh. It is also exceptionally easy to transport and can be reheated or enjoyed cold.

Ingredients

Serves 2

- 1 cup whole-wheat pasta
- 1 (5-ounce) can tuna, washed and drained
- 1/3 cup feta cheese
- 3 cherry tomatoes, cut
- 1 tablespoon olive oil
- 1/4 teaspoon salt
- 1/8 teaspoon ground black pepper

Direction

a. Cook pasta according to the guidance on the container and then drain. Place pasta in a medium bowl.
b. Add tuna and feta cheese to the hot pasta, blending until it starts to dissolve.
c. Add remaining ingredients, blend well, and serve.

Per Serving

- Calories: 438
- Fat: 19g
- Protein: 35g
- Sodium: 881mg
- Fiber: 3g
- Carbohydrates: 32g
- Sugar: 3g

62. Feta and Tuna Pasta Salad

This protein and carb blend is delicious when eaten fresh. It is also exceptionally easy to transport and can be reheated or enjoyed cold.

Ingredients

Serves 2

- 1 cup whole-wheat pasta
- 1 (5-ounce) can tuna, flushed and drained
- ⅓ cup feta cheese
- 3 cherry tomatoes, cut
- 1 tablespoon olive oil ¼ teaspoon salt ⅛ teaspoon ground black pepper

Direction

a. Cook pasta according to the direction on the crate and then drain. Place pasta in a medium bowl.
b. Add tuna and feta cheese to the hot pasta, blending until it starts to dissolve.
c. Add remaining ingredients, mix well, and serve.

Per Serving

- Calories: 438
- Fat: 19g
- Protein: 35g
- Sodium: 881mg
- Fiber: 3g
- Carbohydrates: 32g
- Sugar: 3g

63. High-Protein Tuna Melt

Like a pizza, this open-face sandwich can have all sorts of fixings. Add any ingredients if you'd prefer to vary the recipe.

Ingredients

Serves 1

- 1 whole-wheat English biscuit
- 2 tablespoons tomato sauce or pizza sauce
- 1 (5-ounce) can tuna, drained
- ¼ cup low-fat mozzarella cheese
- 1 teaspoon dried oregano
- ¼ teaspoon garlic salt

Direction

a. Slice biscuit in half and spread tomato sauce on the two halves.
b. Top with tuna, cheese, seasonings, and whatever different fixings you want to add.
c. Place biscuit halves on a pan in the toaster oven or regular oven and sear 2–3 minutes.

Per Serving

- Calories: 412
- Fat: 8g
- Protein: 52g
- Sodium: 1,287mg
- Fiber: 2g
- Carbohydrates: 31g
- Sugar: 3g

64. Lemon Pepper Tilapia

A simple, gentle tasting dish that works out in a good way for anything. Serve over rice or pasta, or enjoy with a side of asparagus or broccoli. You can also sprinkle the fish with olive oil to add more fats to your meal if required.

Ingredients

Serves 4

- (4-ounce) tilapia filets
- 2 tablespoons lemon juice
- ¼ teaspoon lemon pepper seasoning
- ¼ teaspoon garlic salt

Direction

a. Preheat oven to 400°F.
b. Place fish in a 9" × 9" glass baking dish, shower with lemon juice, and add seasonings.
c. Bake 15–20 minutes, or until fish flakes easily.

Per Serving

- Calories: 112
- Fat: 2g
- Protein: 23g
- Sodium: 208mg
- Fiber: 0g
- Carbohydrates: 1g
- Sugar: 0g

65. Shrimp Ceviche

This versatile blend can be presented with chips as a side dish or enjoyed in larger quantities as a

standalone meal.

Ingredients

Serves 2

- ½-pound shrimp, stripped and cooked
- ½ cup diced cherry tomatoes
- ¼ red onion, stripped and cut
- ½ cup finely chopped cilantro
- ½ medium avocado, stripped, pitted, and chopped
- ¼ teaspoon salt
- ⅛ teaspoon ground black pepper 1 large lime

Direction

a. Add shrimp, tomatoes, onion, cilantro, avocado, salt, and pepper to a large bowl and blend well.
b. Cut the lime in half and crush the juices in with the general mish-mash. You can also add slices of lime for extra flavor.
c. Toss the blend well and chill until ready to serve.

Per Serving

- Calories: 222
- Fat: 9g
- Protein: 25g
- Sodium: 469mg
- Fiber: 5g
- Carbohydrates: 12g
- Sugar: 2g

Chapter Eleven: Vegetarian Mains, Sides, and Salads

66. Vegetarian Cakes

This is a without meat alternative to burgers that are easy to make and tastes heavenly. Serve the way you would normally enjoy regular burgers. This can be on a bun, or without anyone else with a side salad.

Ingredients

Serves 4

- 1 (15-ounce) can black beans, drained and washed
- 2 cloves garlic, minced
- 3 tablespoons minced onion
- 1 large whole egg ¼ cup oat bran or ground oats
- ¼ teaspoon salt ⅛ teaspoon ground black pepper

Direction

a. Blend all ingredients with a blender.
b. Form the blend into 4 equally shaped patties.
c. Cook in a medium skillet sprayed with cooking spray over medium heat about 4 minutes for every side.

Per Serving

- Calories: 252
- Fat: 5g

- Protein: 17g
- Sodium: 953mg
- Fiber: 13g
- Carbohydrates: 41g
- Sugar: 5g

67. High-Protein Spread

This is an ideal appetizer or side dish. Present with crackers, chips, or vegetables for plunging.

Ingredients

Serves 2

- ½ cup cottage cheese
- 2 ounces tofu
- 1 tablespoon sun-dried tomatoes
- ½ cup spinach Dash dried basil

Direction

Mix all ingredients in a blender, then serve.

Per Serving

- Calories: 76
- Fat: 3g
- Protein: 8g
- Sodium: 243mg
- Fiber: 1g
- Carbohydrates: 4g
- Sugar: 2g

68. Banana Oatmeal

This take on oatmeal can be eaten with breakfast or filled in as a meal for lunch or supper. It is a fantastic wellspring of carbs, protein, and fiber.

Ingredients

Serves 1

- ½ medium banana, mashed
- ½ cup dry oats
- 1 cup of water
- 4 large egg whites
- 1 (3.5-gram) packet stevia, or other artificial sugar
- ⅛ teaspoon baking powder

Direction

a. Preheat oven to 350°F.
b. In a medium bowl, consolidate all ingredients and blend well. Pour blend into an ovenproof bowl sprayed with cooking spray.
c. Bake 30 minutes, then serve.

Per Serving

- Calories: 282
- Fat: 3g
- Protein: 20g
- Sodium: 290mg
- Fiber: 6g
- Carbohydrates: 45g

- Sugar: 11g

69. Quinoa Burritos

This recipe is a good way of eating quinoa, one of the better total protein sources available on a vegetarian diet.

Ingredients

Serves 2

- 4 large egg whites
- ½ cup cooked quinoa
- ½ cup black beans
- ¼ cup diced red onion
- 2 small whole-wheat tortillas
- ½ cup salsa 1 cup destroyed lettuce
- ½ cup stripped, cubed avocado

Quinoa, the Complete Protein

It's essential to guarantee you are getting finished protein sources with all the amino acids you need on a vegetarian diet. Quinoa is one of the complete protein sources in the plant world, and ought to be a staple in your diet.

Direction

a. Set a medium skillet over average heat, cook egg whites to your desired level of doneness. Expel from heat.
b. Add cooked quinoa, black beans, and onion to the egg whites and mix to join.
c. Spread half the blend on each tortilla.

d. Add salsa, lettuce, and avocado, at that point, fold into burritos and serve.

Per Serving

- Calories: 371
- Fat: 10g
- Protein: 19g
- Sodium: 991mg
- Fiber: 10g
- Carbohydrates: 53g
- Sugar: 6g

70. Zesty Peanut Tempeh Salad

Here's a healthy mix that can be served over greens, eaten as a side dish, or made into a salad.

Ingredients

Serves 2

- 4 ounces tempeh, cut into strips
- 1 cup chopped kale
- 1 tablespoon natural peanut butter
- 1 tablespoon white wine vinegar
- 3 tablespoons water Squeeze ground cayenne pepper Pinch garlic powder

Direction

   a. Place a large pan over medium heat, cook tempeh strips, and kale about 3–4 minutes or until tempeh starts to look brilliant.
   b. Add peanut butter, vinegar, water, cayenne, and garlic powder.

c. Blend well until tempeh is coated with the blend. Mix about brief more and then serve.

Per Serving

- Calories: 181
- Fat: 11g
- Protein: 14g
- Sodium: 59mg
- Fiber: 2g
- Carbohydrates: 12g
- Sugar: 1g

71. Baked Eggplant and Bell Pepper

Here is a great side dish to present with your favorite vegetarian meal.

Ingredients

Serves 2

- 1 medium eggplant, cut
- 1 medium green chile pepper, seeded and diced
- 2 celery stalks, cut
- 2 cloves garlic, minced
- 1 teaspoon dried oregano
- ¼ teaspoon salt
- ⅛ teaspoon ground black pepper
- ¼ cup red wine vinegar

Direction

a. Preheat oven to 400°F.
b. Place eggplant, green pepper, and celery in a 13" × 9" glass dish.

c. Sprinkle with minced garlic, oregano, salt, and black pepper.
d. Pour red wine vinegar over the top.
e. Cover dish with aluminum thwarts and bake 30 minutes.

Per Serving
- Calories: 85
- Fat: 1g Protein: 3g
- Sodium: 336mg
- Fiber: 10g
- Carbohydrates: 19g
- Sugar: 8g

72. Zucchini Oven Fries

The ideal side dish or snack for any occasion and goes well with any main protein dish.

Ingredients

Serves 2

- 1 large zucchini
- 1 tablespoon dried oregano
- 1 tablespoon cumin

Direction
a. Preheat oven to 400°F.
b. Cut zucchini into ¼" × 3" sticks (about the size of standard French fries).
c. Arrange zucchini fries on a nonstick baking sheet.
d. In a small bowl, consolidate flavors and then sprinkle over the zucchini fries.

e. Place in oven and cook 15–18 minutes.

Per Serving
- Calories: 46
- Fat: 1g
- Protein: 3g
- Sodium: 18mg
- Fiber: 3g
- Carbohydrates: 7g
- Sugar: 4g

73. Lemon Quinoa

This is an exceptionally refreshing, flavorful way to serve your quinoa. Tasty all alone, or it tends to be joined with tofu or blended greens.

Ingredients

Serves 4
- 2 cups of water
- 1 cup uncooked quinoa
- 1/3 cup finely chopped onion
- 1 tablespoon olive oil
- 1 tablespoon lemon juice
- 1 teaspoon lemon get-up-and-go

Direction
a. Add quinoa and water in a medium pan and heat to the point of boiling.
b. When quinoa is boiling, turn the heat down to medium-low and add the onion.

c. Place the top on the pot, inclining the top to allow steam to escape, and cook until quinoa is delicate and fluid is absorbed, approximately 12–15 minutes.

d. Once quinoa is cooked, mix in olive oil, lemon squeeze, and get-up-and-go.

Per Serving

- Calories: 193
- Fat: 6g Protein: 6g
- Sodium: 7mg
- Fiber: 3g
- Carbohydrates: 29g
- Sugar: 1g

74. Fresh Corn, Pepper, and Avocado Salad

Whenever you make old fashioned corn, put a couple of ears in a safe spot for this fantastic summer salad.

Ingredients

Serves 6

- 3 ears freshly cooked corn
- 1 medium red chime pepper
- 1 medium ready avocado
- 1 jalapeño pepper, minced
- 1 scallion, daintily cut 1 clove garlic, minced
- Juice of 1 fresh lime
- 2 tablespoons olive oil
- ½ teaspoon freshly ground black pepper

Corn Facts

Corn is high in vitamin C, is a great wellspring of both protein and fiber, and contains antioxidants associated with diminished risk of cardiovascular disease and hypertension. It very well may be eaten hot or cold, on the cob or in single portions, and even popped. Corn develops easily in the home garden. Its sweet taste and vibrant shading add flavor, intrigue, and added sustenance to any meal.

Direction

a. Cut the bits from the corn carefully, utilizing a sharp knife—place in a blending bowl.
b. Core and dice the red pepper and strip and bone the avocado. Add to the bowl, along with the jalapeño, cut scallion (white and green parts), and minced garlic.
c. In a medium bowl, whisk the lime squeeze and oil together. Shower over the salad and prepare to coat—season with freshly ground black pepper.
d. Serve instantly or cover and refrigerate until ready to serve.

Per Serving
- Calories: 135
- Fat: 9g
- Protein: 2g
- Sodium: 5mg
- Fiber: 3g
- Carbohydrates: 13g
- Sugar: 2g

75. Southwestern Beet Slaw

This simple salad will make a beet sweetheart out of you! Destroyed beets are joined with carrots, scallions, garlic, cilantro, and a lime vinaigrette. The subsequent salad is inconspicuously sweet, hot, and spectacular.

Ingredients

Serves 6

- 3 small-medium beets
- 3 scallions, cut
- 2 medium carrots, slice
- ¼ cup chopped fresh cilantro
- 2 cloves garlic
- Juice of 2 fresh limes
- 1 teaspoon olive oil
- ½ teaspoon sans salt bean stew seasoning
- ¼ teaspoon freshly ground black pepper

Keep Your Herbs Fresh Longer

It is regularly difficult to make it through a whole bundle of herbs in one sitting. Keep them fresh by putting them away in a glass of water in the refrigerator. Clasp off the closures as required.

Direction

a. Trim and strip the beets, at that point shred. Place into a blending bowl.

b. Add the scallions, carrots, cilantro, and garlic and mix well to join.

c. Add the lime juice, olive oil, stew seasoning, and black pepper in a small bowl and whisk well to join. Pour dressing over the salad and prepare well to coat.

d. Serve instantly or cover and refrigerate until ready to serve.

Per Serving

- Calories: 38
- Fat: 1g Protein: 1g
- Sodium: 46mg
- Fiber: 2g
- Carbohydrates: 7g
- Sugar: 4g

76. Bean Salad with Orange Vinaigrette

This three-bean salad has citrus contort and is most appropriate for a high-carb day. Canned beans make this a snap to prepare; substitute 1 3/4 cups of each sort of beans if you make them yourself.

Ingredients

Serves 6

- 1 (15-ounce) can no-salt-added kidney beans
- 1 (15-ounce) can no-salt-added garbanzo beans
- 1 (15-ounce) can no-salt-added pinto beans
- 2 shallots, chopped
- 1 medium carrot, destroyed
- 1 small ringer pepper, diced
- 1 small stalk celery, diced

- ¼ cup unadulterated maple syrup
- ⅓ cup apple juice vinegar
- 2 tablespoons freshly pressed orange juice
- 1 tablespoon olive oil
- 1 teaspoon grated orange pizzazz
- ½ teaspoon freshly ground black pepper

Direction
   a. Drain and flush all the canned beans, at that point, place in a blending bowl.
   b. Add the chopped shallot, destroyed carrot, chime pepper, and celery and mix to consolidate.
   c. Place the remaining ingredients into a small blending bowl and whisk well. Pour the dressing over the salad and prepare to coat.
   d. Serve instantly or cover and refrigerate until ready to serve.

Per Serving
- Calories: 393
- Fat: 5g Protein: 19g
- Sodium: 70mg
- Fiber: 16g
- Carbohydrates: 69g
- Sugar: 13g

77. Basic Autumn Salad

A tasty combination of red leaf lettuce, red onion, organic product, and walnuts in a light and tangy vinaigrette. This salad has a moderate amount of carbs so that it could fit a high-or low-carb day.

Ingredients

Serves 4

- 1 large head red leaf lettuce 1 pear, daintily cut
- ½ small red onion, daintily cut
- ½ cup dried black strategic, chopped
- 1 clove garlic, minced
- ⅓ cup chopped walnuts
- 2 tablespoons white balsamic vinegar
- 2 tablespoons olive oil
- ¼ teaspoon freshly ground black pepper

Stock Up and Save

There's nothing more irritating than coming up short on a crucial fix when you're ready to cook. This goes when you're crunched for time or don't have the advantage of requesting. By purchasing things in mass, you'll not exclusively be saving cash, according to unit costs are regularly cheaper, you'll also be supporting against future burden.

Direction

a. Wash the lettuce, pat dry, at that point tear into scaled-down pieces—place in a bowl with the cut pear, onion, figs, and walnuts. Put in a safe spot.

b. Add the vinegar, oil, garlic, and black pepper in a small dish and whisk well to consolidate. Pour the dressing over the salad and prepare to coat. Serve immediately.

Per Serving
- Calories: 224
- Fat: 14g
- Protein: 3g
- Sodium: 29mg
- Fiber: 5g
- Carbohydrates: 25g
- Sugar: 15g

78. Vegetable-Stuffed Poblano Peppers

This lean dish is most appropriate for a high-carb day. Large, unwrinkled poblano peppers work well in this recipe.

Ingredients

Serves 4

- 2 tablespoons olive oil
- minced 2 medium zucchinis, cubed
- 4 cloves garlic, minced
- 1 medium onion, minced
- 2 chipotle chilies in adobo sauce,
- 1½ cups fresh corn parts
- ¾ cup defrosted, drained,
- chopped spinach

- 4 large poblano peppers
- 1 (28-ounce) can squashed tomatoes

Direction
a. Preheat oven to 350°F.
b. Heat oil in a skillet. Add the garlic and onion. Sauté until the onion is softened, then add the chipotle chilies, zucchini, and corn. Sauté until the zucchini starts to soften, about 5–10 minutes. Empty blend into a bowl and mix in the spinach.
c. Slice the poblanos down the center but not all the way through, to shape a pocket. Fill each with the vegetable blend.
d. Pour half of the tomatoes on the base of an 8" × 8" baking dish. Arrange the peppers open-side up in a solitary column—shower with remaining tomatoes.
e. Bake for close to 20 minutes or until cooked through.

Per Serving
- Calories: 221
- Fat: 8g
- Protein: 7g
- Sodium: 32mg
- Fiber: 8g
- Carbohydrates: 36g
- Sugar: 15g

79. Portobello Tacos

Meaty portobellos concoct rapidly, making this a great weeknight meal.

Ingredients

Serves 6

- 8 portobello mushroom caps
- 1 tablespoon olive oil
- 6 (8") corn tortillas 1
- 16 ounces cherry tomatoes, halved
- 1 cup chopped romaine lettuce
- ⅔ cup destroyed red cabbage
- ¼ cup diced onion
- 1 medium avocado, cut
- ½ cup sharp cream

Mushroom By Any Other Name

Agaricus bisporus, when mature, is the portobello mushroom. However, before it gets to that point, it is called cremini, baby bella, champignon, button mushroom, Italian earthy colored, Swiss earthy colored, or Roman mushroom. The name generally relies upon the shade of the cap.

Direction

a. Brush each mushroom cap with oil. Heat a nonstick flame broil pan over medium heat. Barbecue the mushrooms until warmed through, about 3–5 minutes. Cut into ¼"- thick slices.

b. Evenly gap the mushrooms onto the tortillas. Heap the remaining ingredients on the mushrooms. Serve immediately.

Per Serving
- Calories: 211
- Fat: 12g
- Protein: 6g
- Sodium: 45mg
- Fiber: 7g
- Carbohydrates: 24g
- Sugar: 6g

CHAPTER TWELVE: VEGAN MAINS, SIDES, AND SALADS

80. Vegetable Stew with Cornmeal Dumplings

The naturally without gluten cornmeal dumplings consummately supplement the fall vegetables in this hearty stew, making it a total meal in one pot.

Ingredients

Serves 6

- 1 teaspoon olive oil
- 3 chestnut potatoes, stripped and diced
- 3 medium carrots, stripped and cut into ½" pieces
- 2 medium stalks celery, diced
- 1 medium onion, stripped and diced
- 2 rutabagas or turnips, stripped and diced
- cup cauliflower florets
- 2 quarts low-sodium vegetable stock
- 1 tablespoon fresh thyme
- 1 tablespoon fresh parsley
- ⅔ cup water
- 2 tablespoons canola oil
- ½ cup cornmeal
- 2 teaspoons baking powder

- ½ teaspoon salt

Herbivore versus Omnivore

To make this a non-vegetarian, non-vegan meal, use meat stock instead of vegetable stock and add 1 pound of diced, cooked stew hamburger to the vegetables.

Direction

a. Heat olive oil in a non-stick skillet under low heat. Add all vegetables. Sauté until onions are soft and translucent, about 3–5 minutes. Add to a 4-quart slow cooker.

b. Add stock, thyme, and parsley. Mix. Cook up to 4–6 hours on high or 8 hours on low heat until the vegetables are fork-delicate. Mix.

c. In a medium bowl, blend water, oil, cornmeal, baking powder, and salt—Drop-in ¼-cup hills on the stew in a solitary layer. Spread and cook on high 20 minutes without lifting the cover. The dumplings will look soft and light when completely cooked.

Per Serving
- Calories: 204
- Fat: 6g
- Protein: 4g
- Sodium: 436mg
- Fiber: 6g
- Carbohydrates: 35g
- Sugar: 6g

81. Red Beans and Rice

You can add lift to the flavor of this dish by subbing zesty tomato-vegetable juice for the stock or water.

Ingredients

Serves 6

- 1 tablespoon olive oil
- 1 cup changed over long-grain rice
- 1 (15-ounce) can of red beans, drained and washed
- 1 (15-ounce) can of pinto beans, already rinsed and drained
- ½ teaspoon salt
- 1 teaspoon Italian seasoning
- ½ tablespoon dried onion flakes
- 1¼ cups sans gluten vegetable stock or water
- 1 (15-ounce) can diced tomatoes

Herbs and Spices

Individuals regularly mistake herbs for flavors. Herbs are green and are the leaves of plants—the main herb (in Western cooking) that is a flower is a lavender. Now and again, utilized herbs incorporate parsley, basil, oregano, thyme, rosemary, mint, and Italian seasoning blend. Flavors are roots, tubers, barks, or berries; these incorporate pepper, cinnamon, nutmeg, allspice, cumin, turmeric, ginger, cardamom, and coriander.

Direction

a. Lubricate a 4-quart slow cooker with non-stick spray. Add oil and rice; mix to coat the rice in oil.

b. Add red beans, pinto beans, salt, Italian seasoning, onion flakes, tomatoes, and vegetable stock or water to the slow cooker.

c. Mix to consolidate. Spread and cook on low 6 hours or until the rice is delicate.

Per Serving

- Calories: 442
- Fat: 4g Protein: 21g
- Sodium: 422mg
- Fiber: 18g
- Carbohydrates: 83g
- Sugar: 8g

82. Mediterranean Chickpea Bake

This is a delicious meal and can be enjoyed as a side dish or as a main course.

Ingredients

Serves 4

- 5 tablespoons olive oil
- 1 large onion, stripped and finely chopped
- 4 cloves garlic, minced
- 1 large tomato, chopped
- 2 teaspoons ground cumin
- 1 teaspoon paprika
- 2 large bundles fresh spinach, washed
- 2 cups cooked chickpeas
- ¼ teaspoon salt
- ¼ teaspoon pepper

All-Natural Olive Oil Spray

Make your olive oil spray, purchase a clean spray bottle at a hardware store, and fill it with olive oil. If you utilize a spray bottle that you have at home, make sure it has contained nothing that could leave a harmful buildup. Utilize this spray as an alternative to nonstick sprays that don't taste like olive oil.

Direction

a. Place a saucepan over medium heat then heat the olive oil
b. Fry onion and garlic 2–3 minutes until the onion starts to get translucent; at that point, add tomato, cumin, and paprika. Keep cooking for 5 minutes.
c. Add spinach and chickpeas to the pan.
d. Reduce the heat and spread it with a top. Cook, blending much of the time until spinach is withered and chickpeas are delicate. Add salt and pepper to taste.

Per Serving
- Calories: 352
- Fat: 20g
- Protein: 13g
- Sodium: 587mg
- Fiber: 9g
- Carbohydrates: 35g
- Sugar: 5g

83. Smaller than expected Vegetable Burgers

These are very good and are easy to make. On low-carb days, wrap them in romaine lettuce or cabbage leaves, or fill in as-is. On higher-carb days, these are fantastic when stuffed in a pita pocket with tomatoes, lettuce, and cut onion.

Ingredients

Serves 4

- 1 (13-ounce) can red kidney beans, drained and washed
- 1/2 cup dried without gluten bread pieces or squashed tortilla chips (more if beans are exceptionally wet)
- 1/2 cup chopped red onion
- 2 tablespoons barbecue sauce
- 1 large egg
- 1 teaspoon oregano, rosemary, thyme, basil, or sage
- 1/4 teaspoon salt 1/4 teaspoon pepper
- 1/2 cup cooked earthy colored rice
- 2 tablespoons olive oil

The Praises of Brown Rice

In contrast to white rice, which is rice with its external layers evacuated, earthy colored rice has lost just the grain's hard-external body when it gets to the store. Subsequently, some prefer this variety to its increasingly handled relative. Also, the fiber in earthy colored rice may decrease your risk for colon cancer and can help lower cholesterol!

Direction

a. Pulse all ingredients, except rice and canola oil, in a food processor or on the other hand blender. Transform into a medium bowl.

b. Add earthy colored rice to the bean blend.

c. Form the blend into smaller than normal burgers. Heat oil to 300°F and broil the burgers until they are hot.

Per Serving
- Calories: 251
- Fat: 10g
- Protein: 11g
- Sodium: 1,689mg
- Fiber: 8g
- Carbohydrates: 34g
- Sugar: 4g

84. Arugula and Fennel Salad with Pomegranate

Pomegranates pack a high portion of beneficial health-advancing antioxidants. They are in peak season l.e from October through January; you can also substitute dried cranberries.

Ingredients

Serves 4
- 2 large navel oranges
- 1 large pomegranate
- 4 cups arugula
- 1 cup meagerly cut fennel 4 tablespoons olive oil
- ¼ teaspoon salt
- ¼ teaspoon pepper

Fennel Facts

Fennel, a crunchy and marginally sweet vegetable, is a popular Mediterranean fixing. Fennel has a white or greenish-white bulb and long stalks with feathery green leaves coming from the top. Fennel is firmly related to cilantro, dill, carrots, and parsley.

Direction

a. Cut the tops and bottoms off oranges and then remove the remaining strip. Cut each orange into 10–12 small pieces.
b. Remove seeds from the pomegranate.
c. Place orange pieces, arugula, pomegranate seeds, and fennel slices into a large bowl.
d. Coat the salad with olive oil and season with salt and pepper as desired.

Per Serving

- Calories: 224
- Fat: 15g Protein: 3g
- Sodium: 609mg Fiber: 3g
- Carbohydrates: 24g
- Sugar: 15g

84. Apple Coleslaw

This coleslaw recipe is a refreshing, sweet alternative to traditional coleslaw with mayonnaise. Additionally, the sesame seeds give it a pleasant, nutty flavor.

Ingredients

Serves 4

- 2 cups packaged coleslaw blend
- 1 large unpeeled tart apple, chopped
- ½ cup chopped celery
- ½ cup chopped green chime pepper

- ¼ cup flaxseed oil 2 tablespoons lemon juice
- 1 teaspoon sesame seeds

Seeds versus Nuts

Nuts have a higher omega-6 to omega-3 ratio. Seeds, then again, have a vastly different profile. Seeds have a lower saturated-fat substance and are all the more easily digested by individuals with intestinal issues.

Direction
  a. In a medium bowl, consolidate coleslaw blend, apple, celery, and green enthusiasm per.
  b. In a small bowl, whisk the remaining ingredients. Pour over coleslaw blend and hurl to coat.

Per Serving
- Calories: 158
- Fat: 14g
- Protein: 1g
- Sodium: 20mg
- Fiber: 3g
- Carbohydrates: 9g
- Sugar: 3g

85. Root Vegetable Salad

This root salad has a pleasant surface and shading. It will work out in a good way for any traditional fall or winter dish and will make your home smell like a holiday meal.

Ingredients

Serves 4

- 1 medium rutabaga, stripped and cubed
- 1 medium turnip, stripped and cubed
- 6 medium parsnips, stripped and cubed
- 3 tablespoons olive oil
- 1 tablespoon cinnamon
- 3 cloves garlic, chopped
- 1 tablespoon ground ginger
- 1 teaspoon ground black pepper

Root Vegetables

Roots are under-appreciated parts of plants. These underground vegetables are fantastically tasty and are suggested as a part of a balanced diet; they are high in vitamin An and are a pleasant type of carbohydrate fuel, particularly after working out.

Direction

a. Preheat oven to 400°F.
b. Place rutabaga, turnip, and parsnips in a roasting pan and sprinkle with olive oil.
c. Sprinkle with cinnamon, garlic, ginger, and pepper.
d. Toss in the pan to coat and roast 40–50 minutes or until a toothpick slides easily through the vegetables.

Per Serving
- Calories: 247
- Fat: 11g
- Protein: 4g
- Sodium: 79mg
- Fiber: 11g
- Carbohydrates: 36g
- Sugar: 15g

86. Kale and Sea Vegetables with Orange-Sesame Dressing

This salad is a good appetizer for an Asian-themed meal.

Ingredients

Serves 4
- ¼ cup wakame seaweed
- ½ cup sea lettuce 3 cups kale
- ½ teaspoon lemon juice
- ¼ cup fresh-pressed orange juice
- 6 table-spoons in addition to 1 teaspoon sesame seeds
- 1 tablespoon kelp powder

Sea Vegetables

Sea vegetables are among the most nutritious, delicious, and mineral-rich foods on Earth. Ocean water contains all the mineral components known to humans. For example, both kelp and dulse, different kinds of seaweed, are exceeding expectations loaned wellsprings of iodine, which is an essential supplement missing in many diets. Sea vegetables are dried and ought to be reconstituted by soaking them in water before eating.

Direction
   a. Soak wakame and sea lettuce in water 30 minutes. Flush vegetables and discard the water.
   b. Remove stems from the kale. Fold kale leaves and slash into small pieces.
   c. Sprinkle lemon juice onto the kale and massage it by hand to create a shriveling impact.
   d. Place orange juice, 6 tablespoons of sesame seeds, and kelp powder into a blender and mix until smooth.
   e. Toss dressing with the kale and sea vegetables in a large bowl until well secured. Sprinkle the remaining sesame seeds on top.

Per Serving
- Calories: 90
- Fat: 5g
- Protein: 4g
- Sodium: 64mg
- Fiber: 3g,
- Carbohydrates: 9g
- Sugar: 2g

87. Red Pepper and Fennel Salad

Fennel has a fantastic licorice flavor that mixes pleasantly with nuts. The red pepper adds a flash of shading and a touch of pleasantness to the blend.

Ingredients

Serves 2

- ⅓ cup pine nuts, toasted
- 3 tablespoons sesame seeds, toasted
- 2 tablespoons olive oil
- 1 medium red chile pepper, seeded and halved
- 6 leaves romaine lettuce, sliced
- ½ bulb fennel,
- diced 1 tablespoon walnut oil Juice from 1 medium lime
- ½ teaspoon ground black pepper

Walnut Oil

Walnut oil cannot withstand high heat, so it's ideal for adding it to food that has been cooked or is served raw, for example, a salad. If you decide to cook with walnut oil, utilize a lower flame to avoid consuming it.

Direction

a. Preheat grill.
b. In a medium skillet, sauté pine nuts and sesame seeds in olive oil over medium heat 5 minutes.
c. Grill pepper under the oven until the skin is blackened, and the tissue has softened somewhat, about 5–8 minutes.
d. Place pepper halves in a paper bag to cool somewhat. At the point when sufficiently cool to handle, evacuate the skin and cut the pepper into strips.
e. Combine red pepper slices, lettuce, and fennel in a large salad bowl.

f. Add walnut oil, lime squeeze, and black pepper to taste. Blend dressing well with the salad. Add nut blend and serve.

Per Serving

- Calories: 456
- Fat: 43g
- Protein: 7g
- Sodium: 37mg
- Fiber: 6g,
- Carbohydrates: 17g
- Sugar: 5g

88. Cashew-Zucchini Soup

Cashews make this soup thick and creamy and give a serving of heart-healthy fat.

Ingredients

Serves 4

- 5 medium zucchinis
- 1 large Vidalia onion, stripped and chopped
- 4 cloves garlic, chopped
- ½ teaspoon salt, in addition to additional to taste
- ¼ teaspoon ground black pepper, in addition to adding to taste
- 3 cups vegetable stock
- ½ cup raw cashews
- ½ teaspoon dried tarragon

Cashew Nut Butter

To save time, you may substitute cashew nut butter for the whole raw cashews. Enjoy the extra cashew nut butter as a spread on sandwiches and as a plunge for fresh organic produce. Keep in mind; nut butter is high in calories, so limit the segment size.

Direction

a. Coarsely slash zucchini.
b. Spray a large stewpan with non-stick cooking spray. Combine onion to the pan and cook 5 minutes, until soft and translucent. Add garlic and cook 1 moment. Mix in chopped zucchini, ½ teaspoon salt, and ¼ teaspoon ground pepper, and cook over medium heat, secured, blending occasionally, 5 minutes.
c. Add stock and stew 15 minutes.
d. Add cashews and tarragon. Purée soup in a blender in one to two batches. Fill the blender halfway to avoid consumes from the hot fluid.
e. Return soup to pot; season with additional salt and pepper as desired.

Per Serving

- Calories: 117
- Fat: 8g
- Protein: 6g
- Sodium: 585mg
- Fiber: 3g,
- Carbohydrates: 23g,

- Sugar: 2g

89. Saag Tofu

Saag is a stewed Indian dish made with greens—it's perhaps one of the most popular vegan dishes in Indian food. This recipe features peppery, hearty mustard greens.

Ingredients

Serves 4

- 2 tablespoons canola oil
- 1 medium onion, stripped and daintily cut
- 3 cloves garlic, minced
- 2 green chilies, diced
- 2" handle ginger, finely diced
- 2 teaspoons black mustard seeds
- ½ teaspoon turmeric
- 2 teaspoons garam masala
- ½ teaspoon asafetida
- ½ teaspoon ground cayenne
- 16 ounces mustard greens, chopped
- 1¼ cups extra-firm tofu
- ½ cup water

Sorts of Tofu

Tofu comes in many structures. Dampness rich, smooth tofu has a surface similar to panna cotta. Firm tofu has a springy surface and is rather thick. Extra-firm tofu is considerably firmer and has a greater part of the water expelled.

Direction

- a. Heat oil in a large skillet. Sauté onion, garlic, chilies, and ginger until onions are soft, about 5–10 minutes. Add mustard seeds and let them cook until they start to pop.
- b. Add remaining ingredients and cook until mustard greens wither and tofu is warmed through, about 2–5 minutes.

Per Serving

- Calories: 131
- Fat: 8g
- Protein: 4g
- Sodium: 34mg
- Fiber: 5g,
- Carbohydrates: 14g,
- Sugar: 5g

90. Red Onion and Olive Focaccia

Red onions and olives liven up the flavor of this classic Italian bread.

Ingredients

Serves 12

- 1½ table-spoons active dry yeast
- 2½ cups lukewarm water, isolated use
- 3½ cups flour 6 tablespoons olive oil, isolated use
- ½ tablespoon legitimate salt
- ⅓ cup cut Spanish green olives
- 1 small red onion, stripped and daintily cut

Variations on Focaccia

Pretty much anything can top focaccia. Some combinations incorporate rosemary and sea salt, onions and garlic, or spinach and red pepper. Non-vegan forms frequently incorporate meat and a sprinkle of Parmesan at the finish of the cooking time.

Direction

a. In the bowl of a stand blender, break up yeast in ½ cup lukewarm water.
b. Allow sitting for about 10 minutes.
c. Add flour, 4 tablespoons olive oil, remaining water, and salt. Utilize a batter snare to blend until a soft mixture structure.
d. Remove batter from bowl and structure into a round. Grease a 13" × 9" baking pan. Place batter in pan spread with a tea cloth and allows to rise 1½ hours.
e. Preheat oven to 450°F. Press batter into the pan, reaching all corners. Allow rising an additional 15 minutes.
f. Poke batter with the tip of your fingers to create dimples. Brush with remaining olive oil. Scatter olives and onion over the highest point of the bread.
g. Bake 15 minutes. Serve warm or at room temperature.

Per Serving

- Calories: 202
- Fat: 8g
- Protein: 4g
- Sodium: 329mg
- Fiber: 1g
- Carbohydrates: 29g,
- Sugar: 0g

91. Summer Vegetable Tian

Tian is a French vegetable dish comprising of a variety of daintily cut vegetables framing a casserole.

Ingredients

Serves 4

- 2 tablespoons olive oil
- 3 cloves garlic, minced
- 1 medium onion, stripped and chopped
- 2 medium zucchini, cut
- 2 medium yellow squash, cut
- 3 pounds tomatoes, cut
- 2 tablespoons minced basil
- 2 tablespoons minced oregano
- 1 table-spoon lemon get-up-and-go
- 2 tablespoons lemon juice
- 1/2 teaspoon salt
- 1/2 teaspoon freshly ground black pepper

Variations on a Tian

Tians can be made with any variety of vegetables. Take a stab at utilizing onion slices and eggplant. Or then again meagerly cut bits of potato and winter squash for a winter form.

Direction

a. Heat oil in a large skillet. Include onion and garlic also sauté until onion is translucent, about 5–10 minutes.
b. Scrape garlic and onion blend into a large bowl and add remaining ingredients. Mix until ingredients are equitably distributed.

c. Preheat oven to 400°F.

d. Arrange vegetables in a baking dish, alternating slices of zucchini, yellow squash, and tomatoes. Roast 30 minutes. Serve immediately.

Per Serving
- Calories: 172
- Fat: 8g
- Protein: 6g
- Sodium: 323mg
- Fiber: 7g,
- Carbohydrates: 24g,
- Sugar: 15g

92. Sweet and Spicy Brussels Sprouts

Brussels grows to get a bad rap, but you'll be yearning for more when you prepare this batch of Brussels spun in sweet and zesty flavors.

Ingredients

Serves 2
- 2 cups Brussels grows
- ¾ cup chopped shallots, about 2 large
- 1 medium yellow apple, stripped and minced
- ¼ cup water 2 teaspoons organic maple syrup
- ½ teaspoon red pepper flakes
- 1 teaspoon all-natural sea salt
- 1 teaspoon cracked black pepper

Eat Outside the Box Once a Week

How about lima beans? Tempeh? Pinto beans? Whatever fixing it is that makes you glance at a recipe and flip directly past it, attempt it this week! Think about all the foods you thought you hated as a child but love as an adult. Consider some fresh possibilities, then, go there once seven days and consider how many tasty foods you can attempt throughout the following 52 weeks!

Direction

- In a large skillet over medium heat, consolidate Brussels grows, shallots, and apple with ¼ cup of water.
- Shower maple syrup over the skillet and sprinkle with red pepper flakes. Together until onions and apples are soft, and Brussels grows are fork-delicate, about 8–10 minutes.
- Remove from heat and hurl with sea salt and pepper.

Per Serving
- Calories: 138
- Fat: 1g
- Protein: 5g
- Sodium: 1,198mg
- Fiber: 5g
- Carbohydrates: 32g
- Sugar: 14g

93. Garlicky Chickpeas and Spinach

Flavorful chickpeas are lit up with aromatic garlic and vibrant spinach in this brilliant side dish. It can accompany any vegan meal or act as an entrée completely all alone.

Ingredients

Serves 4

- 1 tablespoon extra-virgin olive oil
- 2 cloves garlic,
- minced 2 cups cooked chickpeas
- 2 cups baby spinach leaves
- 8 ounces disintegrated vegan soft cheese
- 1 teaspoon garlic powder
- 1 teaspoon all-natural sea salt
- 1 teaspoon cracked black pepper

The Mighty Chickpea

You can twofold or significantly increase the nutritional greatness of chickpeas by pairing them with foods that add much greater quality sustenance. To the complex carbohydrates and proteins found in the thick, creamy chickpea, you can add significantly more progressively complex carbs, fiber, essential vitamins and minerals, and antioxidants by adding some vegetables like spinach tomatoes, broccoli, or a variety of other supplement thick foods.

Direction

a. In a large skillet heat, olive oil and minced garlic over medium heat until garlic is brilliant and fragrant, about 1 moment. Add chickpeas and spinach, and sauté until beans are heated through, and spinach is dried, about 2–3 minutes.

b. Add vegan cheese and hurl until dissolved.

c. Remove from heat then add garlic powder, salt, and pepper.

Per Serving
- Calories: 322
- Fat: 17g
- Protein: 18g
- Sodium: 760mg
- Fiber: 7g
- Carbohydrates: 27g,
- Sugar: 5g

Chapter Thirteen Pasta

94. Farfalle with Chicken and Pesto

This dish is a low-fat wellspring of protein and carbs and can be made to accommodate your macros based on the ratio of chicken and pasta you use.

Ingredients

Serves 4

- 8 ounces farfalle
- ½-pound fresh green beans close cut
- ½ cup saved pasta water
- ½ cup decreased fat pesto sauce
- 2 cups scaled-down pieces flame-broiled chicken
- ½ cup pasta water.

Direction

a. Cook pasta according to package directions. Drain and save
b. Place green beans in a small pan add clean water to cover them. Spread and steam over medium heat 8 minutes. Drain.
c. Combine cooked pasta, pesto, saved pasta water, chicken, and green beans in a large bowl and mix to consolidate.

Per Serving

- Calories: 308
- Fat: 10g
- Protein: 27g

- Sodium: 421mg
- Fiber: 5g
- Carbohydrates: 51g
- Sugar: 6g

95. Whole-Wheat Penne with Kale and Cannellini Beans

Another high-carb, low-fat meal. This pasta dish is generally excellent to consume after a workout as it has very low degrees of fat.

Ingredients

Serves 2

- 8 ounces whole-wheat penne
- 2 cloves garlic, minced
- 1-pound kale, chopped
- ¼ teaspoon salt 1 teaspoon red pepper flakes
- 1 (14-ounce) of can cannellini beans, drained and flushed
- ½ cup chicken stock or held pasta water

Direction

a. Cook pasta according to package directions. Drain.
b. Spread an average skillet with non-stick cooking spray and sauté garlic 2 minutes over medium heat.
c. Add kale, salt, and red pepper and sauté about 8 additional minutes, or until kale withers and is delicate.
d. Add beans to kale blend along with stock and cooked pasta, mixing to consolidate. Cook for additional 5to7 minutes or until beans reach the desired degree of softness, and serve.

Per Serving
- Calories: 362

- Fat: 3g
- Protein: 17g
- Sodium: 620mg
- Fiber: 9g
- Carbohydrates: 69g
- Sugar: 3g

96. Baked Ravioli

Too fast and easy to make, for those days when you would prefer not to invest an excessive amount of energy cooking.

Ingredients
Serves 4

- 2 (9-ounce) packages chicken ravioli
- 2 cups thick tomato sauce
- ¼ cup grated part-skim mozzarella cheese

Direction

a. Preheat oven to 350°F. Cook pasta according to package directions, but just until ravioli float to the highest point of the saucepan. Drain.
b. Transfer the pasta back to the pan, then add tomato sauce, blending to coat.
c. Pour pasta blend into a 9" × 9" glass baking dish coated with nonstick cooking spray.
d. Sprinkle with mozzarella cheese. Bake 15 minutes.

Per Serving

- Calories: 166
- Fat: 5g
- Protein: 7g

- Sodium: 1,155mg
- Fiber: 2g
- Carbohydrates: 33g
- Sugar: 8g

97. Broccoli-Basil Pesto and Pasta

A pleasant, veggie-packed change from your regular pesto.

Ingredients

Serves 8

- 3½ cups broccoli florets
- 3 (free) cups fresh basil 3 cloves garlic
- 3 tablespoons olive oil
- ¼ teaspoon salt
- ½ teaspoon white pepper
- ¼ cup grated Parmesan cheese
- 3 tablespoons toasted pine nuts
- 1 tablespoon lemon juice
- 1-pound cooked pasta

How to Toast Pine Nuts

Draw out the best flavor of pine nuts, also known as pignoli nuts, by toasting them. Add them to a dry skillet and warm them over low heat. Watch the nuts intently, so they don't consume.

Direction

a. Put the broccoli in a big pot of boiling water. Boil until delicate, about 10–15 minutes. Utilize a slotted spoon to expel the broccoli into a bowl. Allow cooling quickly.

b. Place the broccoli in a blender or food processor. Add the remaining ingredients except for the pasta. Heartbeat until smooth.

c. Pour pesto sauce over hot or cold pasta.

Per Serving
- Calories: 193
- Fat: 10g
- Protein: 6g
- Sodium: 120mg
- Fiber: 3g
- Carbohydrates: 22g
- Sugar: 1g

98. Chicken and Broccoli Fettuccine

A staple at buffets, chicken, broccoli, and ziti is a great flavor combination. The nutritional issue arises when you consider its heavy cream sauce and white pasta. Light and satisfying, this rendition will leave you stimulated, not feeling overloaded!

Ingredients

Serves 2

- 2 tablespoons olive oil

- 1 teaspoon minced garlic
- 1 cup broccoli florets
- 2 table-spoons clean water
- 1½ cups cooked whole-wheat fettuccine
- 1 boneless, skinless chicken breast
- 1 teaspoon all-natural sea salt

Direction
   a. Prepare a skillet with 1 tablespoon of olive oil then lower the heat.
   b. Cut chicken breast into 1" pieces, and sauté for 2–3 minutes.
   c. Add minced garlic, broccoli, and 1 tablespoon of water to the skillet and keep sautéing for 4–5 minutes.
   d. Add water as expected to prevent staying and advance steaming.
   e. Remove from heat when broccoli is somewhat softened, and the chicken is cooked through with juices running clear.
   f. Toss the chicken and broccoli with the fettuccine and remaining tablespoon of olive oil. Season with the sea salt, and serve immediately.

Per Serving
- Calories: 369
- Fat: 16g
- Protein: 19g
- Sodium: 1,239mg
- Fiber: 3g
- Carbohydrates: 36g

- Sugar: 1g

99. Pepper, Onion, and Shrimp Kebabs

Kebabs aren't only for chicken and steak. This delectable recipe makes a satisfying plate of succulent shrimp and fresh vegetables flame-broiled and seasoned to flawlessness.

Ingredients Serve 2

- 1-pound large shrimp, stripped and deveined
- 1 Vidalia onion, cut into 1" pieces
- 1 small green chile pepper, cut into 1" pieces
- 1 small red ringer pepper, cut into 1" pieces
- 1 small yellow chime pepper, cut into 1" pieces
- 1 tablespoon olive oil
- 2 teaspoons garlic powder
- 1 teaspoon all-natural sea salt
- 1 teaspoon freshly ground black pepper

Direction
 a. Heat a barbecue to medium heat, and prepare sticks.
 b. Spit the shrimp and vegetables in the alternating request.
 c. Paint the speared shrimp and veggies softly with the tablespoon of olive oil, and sprinkle with the flavors.
 d. Grill for 2 to 3 moments on the two side, or until shrimp is pink and cooked through.

Per Serving
- Calories: 367
- Fat: 11g
- Protein: 48g
- Sodium: 1,520mg
- Fiber: 5g
- Carbohydrates: 18g
- Sugar: 7g

Chapter Fourteen; Soups

100. Corn and Black Bean Chili

Most bean stew takes all day to cook, but this recipe has just a couple of ingredients and is ready rapidly.

Ingredients

Serves 4

- 1-pound lean ground hamburger
- 2 teaspoons bean stew powder
- 1 (14-ounce) package solidified corn and beans mix
- 1 (14-ounce) can low-sodium hamburger stock
- 1 (14-ounce) can season tomato sauce

Direction

a. Combine ground hamburger and bean stew powder in a large Dutch oven. Cook 6 minutes on medium or high heat or until hamburger is seared, mixing to disintegrate. Drain and come back to the pan.

b. Stir in solidified corn blend, stock, and tomato sauce; heat to the point of boiling.

c. Cover, diminish heat and stew 10 minutes.

d. Uncover and stew 5 minutes, occasionally mixing, at that point serve.

Per Serving

- Calories: 273

- Fat: 7g
- Protein: 30g
- Sodium: 922mg
- Fiber: 4g
- Carbohydrates: 26g
- Sugar: 4g

101. Creamy Corn Chowder

Many people don't consider chowder being the healthiest or most calorie-aware of meal choices, but this recipe breaks the form. It's packed with delightful, all-natural ingredients specifically picked for their sustenance and taste.

Ingredients

Serves 6

- 6 cups almond milk, isolated
- 1 cup potatoes, stripped and chopped
- 1 cup carrots, chopped
- 4 cups bit corn
- 1 teaspoon all-natural sea salt
- 1 cup low-fat plain Greek yogurt

Direction

a. In a large pot over medium heat, measure 3 cups of the almond milk, potatoes, and carrots then allow boiling. Lessen heat to low and stew for 10 minutes.

b. Add kernel corn, add remaining 3 cups almond milk, and salt, and stew for another 5–8 minutes.

c. Remove the soup from the gas and let it cool for about 5 minutes.

d. Slowly blend in the Greek yogurt ¼ cup at a period until well mixed.

Per Serving
- Calories: 116
- Fat: 0.3g
- Protein: 7g
- Sodium: 608mg
- Fiber: 3g
- Carbohydrates: 14g
- Sugar: 4g

102. Pumpkin Soup Base

This soup is intended to be cooked in large amounts and then put away solidified for later use. After reheating, it is sweet as is, or you can add vegetables, nuts, or anything else you like.

Ingredients

Serves 6
- 4 medium onions, stripped and chopped
- 4 stalks celery, chopped
- 3 cloves garlic, minced
- 2 tablespoons olive oil
- 1-pound raw pumpkin, stripped, seeds expelled, chopped
- 8 cups chicken stock, or more if required

Direction
a. Cook onions, celery, and garlic in a large saucepan over medium heat with the oil until vegetables are soft, around 5 minutes.

b. Add pumpkin and enough stock to reach the highest point of the pumpkin simply.
c. Bring blend to a boil while mixing; at that point, decrease the heat and stew 40 minutes.
d. Blend this softened blend in batches in a blender or food processor until smooth (being careful not to consume yourself with the hot fluid). Utilize immediately or freeze for later use.

Per Serving
- Calories: 210
- Fat: 9g
- Protein: 10g
- Sodium: 483mg
- Fiber: 2g
- Carbohydrates: 24g
- Sugar: 10g

103. Sweet and Spicy Carrot Soup

Sweet carrots get significantly better as they stew in their juices. Spiced up with ginger and shallots, the carrots take on a profundity of flavor that makes this soup ideal.

Ingredients Serve 4
- 2 table-spoons ginger, grated
- 2 shallots, minced
- 4 cups water 1-pound baby carrots
- ¼ teaspoon cayenne pepper

Bigger Batches Save Time: Rather than single out meals according to what ingredients you have (or don't have!) on hand, you can simplify your meal prep by having large batches of certain staples ready to go in your freezer. Stocks, soups, and sauces that save well can be made in large quantities, put away in glass containers, and solidified for quite a long time, making meal prep as straightforward as defrosting while at work or play.

Direction

a. In a pot over medium heat, consolidate the ginger and shallots with ¼ cup of the water. Sauté for 4–5 minutes, or until shallots are soft and translucent.

b. Add remaining water, carrots, and cayenne pepper to the pot and bring to a boil. Cover and diminish heat to low.

c. Simmer for up to 30 to 45 minutes or until carrots are fork-soft. Expel from heat.

d. Using a submersion blender, emulsify until the desired thickness is achieved.

Per Serving

- Calories: 48
- Fat: 2g
- Protein: 1g
- Sodium: 88mg
- Fiber: 4g
- Carbohydrates: 11g,
- sugar 5g

Desserts

104. Peanut Butter Protein Cookies

The protein and fat in this recipe will keep you full with minimal carbohydrates. This is an ideal treat for low-carb days.

Ingredients Serve 10

- 1 cup peanut butter
- 2 large egg whites
- 1 scoop vanilla protein powder
- ¾ cup stevia
- 1 teaspoon cinnamon.

Direction
  a. Preheat oven to 350°F.
  b. Set all ingredients in a small dish and mix to consolidate.
  c. Shape batter into 2" balls and place on greased treat sheet.
  d. Bake for 10 minutes.

Per Serving

- Calories: 192
- Fat: 13g
- Protein: 10g
- Sodium: 133mg
- Fiber: 2g
- Carbohydrates: 12g
- Sugar: 10g

105. Oatmeal Protein Cookies

These treats are higher in carbs and protein with exceptionally low fat. The oatmeal also gives fiber, which will help keep you feeling full.

Ingredients

Serves 7

- 1¾ cup oats
- 4 scoops vanilla protein powder
- ½ cup applesauce
- ½ cup egg whites
- 1 tablespoon olive oil
- 1 tablespoon stevia Dash cinnamon

Direction

a. Preheat oven to 350°F.
b. Set all ingredients in a big bowl and mix to blend.
c. Shape mixture into 2" balls, and place on greased treat sheet.
d. Bake 10–15 minutes.

Per Serving

- Calories: 170
- Fat: 3g
- Protein: 19g
- Sodium: 53mg
- Fiber: 2g
- Carbohydrates: 17g
- Sugar: 3g

106. Protein Cheesecake

This recipe can be modified with any organic product or fixings you want to add, but it stands fine all alone. Utilize without fat cream cheese to hold calories in line.

Ingredients Serve 8

- 24 ounces sans fat cream cheese
- 2 scoops vanilla whey protein powder
- ¾ cup stevia 1 teaspoon vanilla extract
- 3 large whole eggs
- 1 tablespoon lemon juice

Direction
a. Preheat oven to 350°F.
b. Set all ingredients in a big dish and blend in with hand blender.
c. Pour blend into a pie pan coated with nonstick cooking spray.
d. Bake 45 minutes. Expel from oven and refrigerate 3 hours or until ready to serve.

Per Serving
- Calories: 137
- Fat: 4g
- Protein: 20g
- Sodium: 501mg
- Fiber: 0g
- Carbohydrates: 5g

- Sugar: 3g

107. Peanut Butter Banana Frozen Greek Yogurt

This dish rushes to prepare and makes a well-adjusted sweet that contains protein, carbs, and fat.

Ingredients Serve 1

- ½ cup nonfat plain Greek yogurt
- 1 medium solidified banana, cut
- 2 tablespoons peanut butter

Direction

Combine all ingredients together and blend in a blender until smooth, and serve immediately.

Per Serving

- Calories: 342
- Fat: 17g
- Protein: 14g
- Sodium: 215mg
- Fiber: 5g
- Carbohydrates: 42g
- Sugar: 26g

108. Cinnamon-Pear Frozen Yogurt

This delectable, fall-roused solidified yogurt is high in carbs and makes the ideal sweet for your high-carbohydrate days.

Ingredients

Serves 2

- 1 (15-ounce) can pear halves

- 2 cups low-fat vanilla yogurt
- 2 tablespoons stevia
- ½ teaspoon cinnamon
- ¼ teaspoon allspice

Direction

- Drain pears, saving ½ cup of the juice.
- Place pears in a blender or food processor and purée.
- Add remaining ingredients and saved pear juice to the blender, mix until smooth, and freeze until ready to serve. You can also combine the ingredients to a frozen yogurt maker if you have one.

Per Serving

- Calories: 365
- Fat: 3g
- Protein: 13g
- Sodium: 172mg
- Fiber: 6g
- Carbohydrates: 74g
- Sugar: 68g

Conclusion

Carb cycling is a great way to get in shape. You get the opportunity to eat your favorite foods, stay fueled up and stimulated for the day, and learn to make insightful eating choices that will help support your body's natural potentials. Whether you want to create lean and strong muscles or simply want to maintain a healthy weight, carb cycling can be the diet program for you. All it takes is determination, compliance with some rules, and your eyes concentrated on the goals. Stay empowered, stay happy, and stay healthy with carb cycling!

CPSIA information can be obtained
at www.ICGtesting.com
Printed in the USA
BVHW041520201120
593806BV00012B/1185